Heart Attack
and
Back

A Story of Denial

Steven A. Jaynes

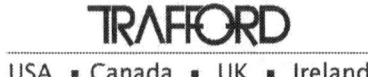
TRAFFORD
USA ▪ Canada ▪ UK ▪ Ireland

Note for Librarians: A cataloguing record for this book is available from Library and Archives
Canada at www.collectionscanada.ca/amicus/index-e.html
ISBN 1-4120-5258-0

Edited by Patti Sculley-Lane

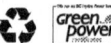

*Printed on paper with minimum 30% recycled fibre. Trafford's print shop
runs on "green energy" from solar, wind and other environmentally-friendly power sources.*

TRAFFORD

Offices in Canada, USA, Ireland and UK
This book was published *on-demand* in cooperation with Trafford Publishing. On-demand
publishing is a unique process and service of making a book available for retail sale to the
public taking advantage of on-demand manufacturing and Internet marketing. On-demand
publishing includes promotions, retail sales, manufacturing, order fulfilment, accounting and
collecting royalties on behalf of the author.

Book sales for North America and international:
Trafford Publishing, 6E–2333 Government St.,
Victoria, BC v8t 4p4 CANADA
phone 250 383 6864 (toll-free 1 888 232 4444)
fax 250 383 6804; email to orders@trafford.com
Book sales in Europe:
Trafford Publishing (uk) Ltd., Enterprise House, Wistaston Road Business Centre,
Wistaston Road, Crewe, Cheshire cw2 7rp UNITED KINGDOM
phone 01270 251 396 (local rate 0845 230 9601)
facsimile 01270 254 983; orders.uk@trafford.com
Order online at:
trafford.com/05-0153

10 9 8 7 6 5 4 3 2 1

TABLE OF CONTENTS

INTRODUCTION

Fear and Denial

When people ask me about my experience, which happens frequently and is the reason for writing this book, I know their questions before they ask. When I start to explain why I think I had the attack, I can see familiarity in their eyes. Sometimes I get the feeling from folks inquiring about my experience that they don't really want me to answer. It seems they would be more comfortable if they could cover their eyes and peek at me through their fingers! I understand that heart attacks do not make for pleasant conversation. This is actually the beginning of denial. "Won't happen to me!"

As you read my story, you will come to understand how denial almost killed me. It is actually a more common phenomenon than one may think. Denial kills over a quarter of a million people yearly.

Deep down inside, we all relate to each other. It is important to understand that we are all susceptible to cardiac problems. This fear is a huge problem. Denial is the enemy. Fast, quick professional treatment is available, and will save lives.

As you read on, I will take you through the process (mine at any rate) of the emergency room experience, diagnostics and how the doctors see it, the events leading up to my surgery and then the surgery itself. I am not going to try to explain the actual operation! But rather how I felt, how the hospital experience went, and some of the characters involved.

My hope is that you will find this book informative and entertaining. However, if I can help one person to face reality, instead of going into denial when they experience cardiac difficulty, this book will be a success!

There are approximately 1.1 million heart attacks every year in this country. One third end in fatality, primarily due to denial. The sooner a cardiac victim gets medical help, the less severe and less life threatening the attack can be.

Please visit my web site http://www.heartattackandback.com for more information about me, this book and fighting denial.

Prolog

7am Monday Morning November 15, 1998

The regular crowd was working out, and the little conversations that weave in and out of a gym in between sets were typical of a Monday morning. Quiet after two days off, people were just getting up to speed, spotting each other and telling stories of the weekend while waiting to recover before starting another set.

I had just finished a great chest workout and was about to do some cardio. Stepping up onto the cardio deck, I began to power up a treadmill when, suddenly, I felt like I had just run out of gas. Not the tired but satisfied feeling you get after any great exercise. Just plain out of gas!

For the first time in my many years of five day a week workouts, I went to a chair by the trainer's corner and sat down. After a short while one of the staff, a trainer named Chris that I had known for a few years, came over and asked if I was OK?

"Oh yeah," I said, "just a little tired."

"I've never seen you look so pale," he continued. "I'm a little concerned you may be having some trouble."

"Don't be silly!" I said. "I'm fine."

I sat there for twenty minutes. Another trainer came over and said, "You look like shit!"

I wasn't feeling any better, but I had a lot to do that day and wanted to get on with my agenda. So off to the showers I went. I made it to the locker room but had to sit down again. This was frustrating for a guy who was used to running three to five miles three or four times a week.

I began to get concerned. That was when another friend, Abdel, a big Moroccan Trainer, came to me with the following information;

"The last guy I see like this," he said in his heavily accented English," was dead ten minutes later!"

"Great," I replied.

I was still sitting on the bench in the locker room, digesting what Abdel had told me, when Doug, another friend came walking in. Doug is a local detective who is without doubt one of the funniest men I have ever had the pleasure of knowing. A great cop, he is a former football player and looks the part. Huge, meaty arms and wide shoulders, his presence is at once commanding and intimidating, until he opens his mouth that is, and something outrageously funny comes out.

"Now, listen to me very carefully," he began in his customary way. "Right now it is very early on Monday morning, I'm am CPR certified and would be legally bound to resuscitate you if you go down. I am not, repeat not, going to suck face with you this morning. I have just called 911 and they are on their way. So just sit still and get used to it, boy-o!"

Sometimes, events seem to take on a life of their own. I felt like a passenger on an out of control bus, or an observer of someone else's life. This was me they were talking about, 911 for me! Shit!

At this point, it was quite evident that everyone was thinking heart attack. But not me! I don't know what I did think, but a heart attack was something that happened to other people. Don't they always get a pain in the jaw or shooting pain down their arm? I was feeling none of that, no pain in my chest, no shortness of breath. So I sat and waited for the rescue crew, feeling silly, and at the same time wondering why I felt so unreal.

The firemen and rescue folks didn't give me too much time to wonder. They arrived in minutes and slapped a measuring device on me that confirmed: HEART ATTACK, BIG ONE!

All I could think to myself was, "Cut the shit, I don't have time for this!" But reality comes screaming in when they lay you on the stretcher and head for the door.

As they wheeled me out, I said to my buddy Joe, "Call my wife, Laura and tell her what's going on. But don't freak her out!"

CHAPTER ONE

Family History

After the initial shock of having a life altering experience, the natural train of thought is, "Why?"

At the time I was a typical American male, 47 years old with a job, family and regular life. For years I had been careful of what I ate. I had quit drinking and smoking and had been in a regular exercise program for years. So what happened?

Reflecting on my history, I had all the ingredients for cardiac arrest. When I was young I ate and drank too much, with no regard to fat content or how it affected me. I had spent years in the automobile business, most of them in sales management. In addition to lack of diet and exercise, there was plenty of stress.

My Father had had a stroke many years earlier that was the death of him. Two of his brothers died from massive heart attacks, as well as a sister who died of congestive heart failure. My Mom, who was living with my family at the time, had had a major heart attack at the dinner table one night! That she survived is credited to my wife rushing her to the hospital. The importance of immediate medical assistance in the instance of cardiac arrest cannot be overstated. So heart disease was demonstrably in my family history. Yet I denied any fear that I might be affected.

Laying the Groundwork for Survival

I clearly remember being thirty years old, an overweight smoker and drinker. One day I tried to do some push-ups. I couldn't do one! So I resolved right then and there to do at least one push-up every day. In a short time I was able to do ten. Encouraged, I started to walk. Exercise was a start but I knew I had to do more. I was determined to fulfill my life long goal of quitting cigarettes, the hardest of all the addictions, with the exception of heroin. Motivated by my new enthusiasm, I quit cold turkey. The walking and exercise took the focus off my withdrawal from nicotine. It was difficult. I had stopped and started several times before. But this time I beat my addiction, and have enjoyed the benefits of being smoke free ever since.

At age thirty-six, after discussing my drinking patterns with my doctor, I decided to quit drinking. I had never had a problem with the law; no DWIs, days lost from work due to hangovers, or ugly episodes at home. I was a happy drinker, just drinking too much. My doctor said if I continued with this pattern it could turn me into a hard alcoholic soon. So I quit, and have not had a drink since November fifteenth, 1986.

I had successfully stopped smoking and drinking. My exercise program became my focus. It replaced the kick I had been getting from booze and cigarettes.

I had religiously walked at least five out of seven days a week for several years. I had a route around the lake near my house. I actually started my running training by accident.

One day, I wanted to walk my route, but was running out of time. As sales manager for a local Ford dealership, being on time was an example I had always set. But my walk had become important to me. The rest of the day was for everybody else. This part of the day, this short period of time, was mine. It was for me. So I said, the hell with it, if I was ten minutes late, so be it. It was my health I was thinking about!

My walking route took me across a good-sized field, and in an effort to make up a little time, I decided to run across the field. It actually felt pretty good! I was surprised. I shouldn't have been. I had been walking regularly for a number of years, and my body was ready for more. It was so successful that I decided to run the field every time I walked.

As time passed, I ran across the field regularly. I started to run during additional stretches of my walk. A little here, a little there, and soon it became easier and easier. I started to notice other things. My weight was easier to control. My energy level was greatly increased. Everything seemed better, including my sex life!

My goal became to run the entire route around the lake. And one day, I did just that! I still remember the elation, the pure joy! As I ran the last leg of the route through the woods on a trail that led home, I raised my arms in the air and yelled like Rocky Balboa running up the steps in Rocky! I couldn't contain myself. I was able to run after having been such a sedentary person.

So I became a runner. I read books about running. I would seek out runners and ask them questions. Their answers would motivate me further.

After several years of running in all types of weather (real runners don't let a storm, rain or snow, keep them off the road!) I joined an inexpensive gym ($99.99 per year!) primarily to be able to use a treadmill when the really inclement or hot weather made it difficult to run outside.

After months of running on a treadmill at the gym, the owner started to encourage me to cross train with weights. I did it, somewhat reluctantly. But after a while, I got the bug for lifting as well as running. The cross training paid off. Plus I met a whole new world of like-minded people. I found that I actually would become more motivated and committed to my workout programs being around others whose goals were similar.

The routine of lifting and running was something I continued and still continue. There is no question in my mind that it saved my life.

CHAPTER TWO

Ride To The Emergency Room

The ambulance parked out front. The doors opened like the maw of a monster that was going to swallow me up.

Rescue workers are a special breed, rushing through traffic and risking their own safety to save a stranger's life. My gratitude at this point was overshadowed by what was becoming confused fear. When one of the ambulance staff stated that he was going to start an IV line, I balked.

"Are you refusing treatment?" asked a man dressed like a fireman.

You have to understand, I wasn't even sure they were right, that I was suffering cardiac arrest. I'm not sure what made me deny that my problem was cardiac related, but two things stand out.

First, no one thinks they are really going to have a heart attack. I was 47 – too young to have an attack. Even with a family history of heart related problems, the natural reaction is that a heart attack is so awful, it couldn't happen to me.

Second, I was having none of the popular or best-known symptoms. I just felt like the plug had been pulled. I had no pain in the jaw, pain running down my arm or crushing pressure in my chest. My chest didn't hurt at all. In fact, my chest never felt pain.

I started to answer the medic, but he seemed disgusted at my lack of co-operation and said, "Fine, have it your way," and went up front to sit with the driver.

Even with my extensive sales and customer service background I was taken off guard. I should have realized, medics are just people and they can be offended!

It was about eight o'clock in the morning, and Rt. 101A was a commuter crammed mess. On went the siren! And lights I'm sure.

I thought to myself, "This is really happening to me!"

After a few minutes we were at the highway and traffic was backed up the on-ramp. I could tell by my limited view that the driver was half on the grass, half on the pavement, and trying to pass everyone. Drivers were doing there best to pull over, just as I had for ambulances a hundred times before. The big difference this time was that I was inside!

That's when the pain started. Quickly, my shoulders, the palms of my hands and my feet started to throb with pain. I started to think that an IV line with some morphine in it sounded pretty good now.

"Hey," I said to the medic who was still sitting up front with the driver, "If you want to start that line now it would be OK," I offered, feeling foolish.

"No, we'll wait until we get to the hospital now," he replied.

To this day I'm not sure if I had offended him that badly or if he was just following protocol. I can tell you that I was suddenly in more pain than I had ever felt. The only comparison I can make is to a toothache that is so bad you need a root canal. Only in many places at once!

Finally, we pulled into St. Joseph's hospital in Nashua, NH. Hurried hands pulled my stretcher out and into the emergency room I went. Soon, nurses and doctors surrounded me. IV lines started to sprout from my arms! Morphine flowed like water, but the pain just stayed with me. I had a nurse on each hand, foot, and shoulder, rubbing and trying to get some blood flowing to those spots.

A familiar face walked into the room. The same doctor credited with saving my Mom's life when she was struck with her heart attack was standing over me! I immediately felt reassured and somewhat comforted.

After examining me, the doctor offered this rather sobering assessment, "Steve, I think I should tell you that there is a very good possibility that you won't survive this heart attack!"

No, my life did not flash before my eyes. But it did cause me to think!

"What are you saying doc, I got five minutes to get good with GOD?" I replied.

He smiled at my bravado but didn't reply. After several minutes of doctoring I asked, "So, what do you think doc, is there a God?"

I have my own thoughts and beliefs about theology and am not sure why I asked; I guess it was just nervous conversation.

He answered with a question, "What do you think?"

I replied, "Well, right now I'm hoping there is!"

"Yeah," he stated, "there aren't any atheists in the foxhole!"

I Get A Visitor

Some really strange things happen to all of us in life, but timing is everything.

A friend from the gym had convinced his girlfriend to start working out and I had met her there several times. She seemed like a nice girl, and good looking too. She was at the gym that morning. She had seen me taken out of the gym, and had decided to follow the ambulance and see if I was all right.

So, there I was, in the emergency room, contemplating the fact that I might be living my final moments, when in walks this good looking girl. I was glad to see a familiar face. Right then, my wife of thirty years also came walking in. My visitor promptly wished us the best and exited.

My wife then turned to me and said, "So this is how I find out you have another woman in your life!"

Talk about injustice. This was not a girlfriend of mine! Just a concerned acquaintance who probably thought that was what her boyfriend would want her to do! So I just lay there, trying to comprehend all that was transpiring.

The doctor came in just then and asked my wife to leave the room. He had work to do. My wife's questions and my explanations where just going to have to wait. All I could do was go with the flow and hope there would be another time for discussion.

After my wife left, the doctor explained he was going to shoot me up with a new clot-busting drug, just off the shelf, very effective and very expensive. Quite honestly, I couldn't have cared less about the price!

"If this is going to work, it will take about ten minutes," he stated as he injected the drug in one of my IV lines.

At that point, I became determined to live. I had to make sure my wife understood that my visitor was just trying to be helpful and was not anything but an acquaintance of mine from the gym.

I started to concentrate on relaxing, trying to feel my heart, like I had been taught to feel each individual muscle when I was working out. Relax, breath, relax, think positive, visualize myself getting up and walking out the door.

About forty-five minutes later, it worked! I lay there literally feeling the blood rushing into my arms, hands, feet and up to my head. I could physically feel it rushing in! And the pain vanished! Gone! In fact, I felt great!

"It worked!" I said excitedly.

The doctor looked up from the meter he had been studying.

"Just now?" he asked and stated at the same time.

"Yeah," I shot back, "just now. I can feel the blood returning to my arms and feet." I told him I felt good enough to get my clothes on and head home.

"Just lie there and be still," he said, "for the next twenty four hours you are going to be extremely susceptible to stroke or shock."

Now that I could somewhat relax and review my situation, I accepted several concepts that I had been resisting. First, I accepted that I had had a heart attack, and that this would be changing major things in my life, and secondly, I was temporarily out of the woods. It had taken a few hours, but I got my chance to talk to my wife and straighten things out about my attractive visitor.

The Waiting Game

Reality seeped into my consciousness like rainwater into a leaky cellar. I was being wheeled to a room, a room in which to wait for…what?

I had been in the hospital before. I had Pneumonia in my thirties and had been admitted for several nights, recovered and discharged all without so much as a pin prick. Needles terrify me! I almost didn't get married when I heard about the blood test! There I was IV's in each arm, still pretty buzzed on the morphine, and headed for my room! My hospital room! I should have been heading up the highway to work.

The good news was I was hungry, really hungry. Since my attack had come after a complete workout, and cardiac arrest is a very energy draining effort, I shouldn't have been surprised at my appetite. I asked about food and was told that was allowed. And in short order I finished both meals I had ordered.

Satiated, and comfortable in my room, I started to take inventory of my situation.

I noticed a note posted on a bulletin board near my bed. It said, "no venous punctures." I'm not trained to understand what that means, but my aversion to needles made the note a welcome friend. I believe that they pump tons of extra blood out of you whenever they want. I'm convinced that they really have an involuntary blood drive going on 24/7, and they collect it a tube at a time! So when, just as I suspected would happen, a very pretty nurse with a huge needle came into my room, my self-preservation instincts came on full force.

"Hi, I just need to get a little blood," said the nurse as she started to prep a vein.

"I don't think the Doctor wants you to jab me there," I stated, hoping the panic and dread I was really feeling didn't come through.

"I have to get the blood from a fresh source," said the Vampiress.

"Well I think the Doctor wants you to use the IV that I already have going here," I offered hopefully.

"Oh no, we absolutely have to get blood directly from a vein to make sure that none of the medications or anything else contaminates the results," she patiently explained.

Trying not to offend her (remembering the medic in the ambulance) and also not to let my real hand show (fear of the needle) I pointed to the note posted next to my bed.

"What do you suppose that means?" I asked.

Somewhere there is a fine line between fending for yourself and professional pride. I guess I had crossed the line, because now she was visibly agitated. So, in an effort to let her feel back in charge (after all I didn't know how much interaction I was going to have with this particular nurse) I continued that the good Doctor had used one of the new clot busting drugs on me and that was, I was sure, the reason for the note.

This seemed to make sense to her, and the blood was drawn (painlessly I might add) from the existing IV. With that, she assured me that future punctures would be needed as additional requests for my blood were received. Leaving me with that forlorn prediction seemed to satisfy her, although undoubtedly not as much as a good jab would have.

Soon after, Laura was sitting by my bed. We looked at each other in amazement. I was having a hard time accepting that I really was grounded in this room. She was having a very hard time with it all.

"What did the doctor say was going to happen to me?" I asked Laura.

"Some tests. I think they want to see how you are responding to the medications they've given you. I really don't know too much." She finished.

And so the waiting game began in earnest. That was the longest Monday of my life! Over the next several days, my time was filled (or not) with visitors (thank god for visitors) and contemplating my fate. Enough questions to fill a book raced through my and my family's minds.

CHAPTER THREE

Hope Out of Despair

That evening, the first of many wonderful things to come of this rather horrible experience occurred.

I lay in my bed alone, thinking of all the things that I would never do again. The gym and running had been a big part of my life. It was how I controlled my weight, relieved my stress and was a huge social event every day for me.

At the gym I tend to feed off the energy of other people, it motivates me. So the thought of losing all this was weighing heavily on my heart, which had already been hammered that day! Imagine how it seemed when a pleasant looking nurse with red hair and a twinkle in her eye came into my life.

"Hi Steve," she said as if we had known each other for years." How are you feeling?"

"I hope I look better than I feel," I responded, curious now because she was almost smirking.

"My name is Jody, and I'm best friends with your friend Priscilla from the gym!" she began. "She called me today and told me all about you and what happened today. She also told me how you like to work out and run. You must be feeling discouraged about now, is that right honey?"

"I don't know what's going to happed to me," was all I could stammer.

"Well I do. I run the cardiac rehab center here at St. Joe's. When the doctors are done doing what they are going to do, I am going to help you get back to where you want to be, lifting and running again!"

I was floored! Here was this super lady telling me there was light at the end of the tunnel. My feelings of gratitude to her for this optimistic view of the future, and for my friend Priscilla for taking the time to call her and send her to me, were overwhelming. In five short minutes she had taken me from the doldrums of despair to envisioning my old self as a possible future.

When Jody had finished delivering her message of hope, she turned and left the room. I lay there trying to imagine my future. A plan seemed to emerge that might include getting back to normal. It was clear to me that all any one who has been struck down wants is to get back to normal.

My Room!

Time doesn't go quickly when you are waiting to find out the plan set for you. I felt as though my life had been going along a major highway and had just run into a cliff of jello. I was confined to my room with a brief route along the corridors allowed, as long as I towed my IV equipment with me.

I had been in the automobile business for over twenty years, so it was no surprise that one of the night nurses was a former customer of mine. When you are in the hospital waiting for the plan, and there are no visitors, which is most of the time, a friendly face anywhere is huge. And you look for something, anything, familiar. So we chatted, and it helped.

After several days, the gods of the hospital had made a decision. It had been decided that I would travel 20 minutes north by ambulance to Catholic Medical Center (CMC) in Manchester NH at 5:30 AM Friday morning, and have several tests performed upon my person.

The first would be an angiogram. This is a procedure where a catheter is introduced into your vein and artery system through a puncture in the thigh.

I thought, "Great, here we go with the really heavy stuff, punctures from hell and who knows what else!"

After that, barring unforeseen consequences, an angioplasty would be performed. The angiogram would show the doctor exactly what artery needed clearing or opening.

The doctor briefly assured me that all would be well, that CMC was one of the leading cardio-thoracic centers in the world, and I would be on my way to Jody in rehab in no time.

This all sounded pretty good. But as the day wore on, I began to imagine the process in my mind. Drilling into my thigh with a tube, up my veins and arteries to my heart! Soon, the tube was the size of my lawn hose! I began to take frequent trips, my IV in tow, up and down the corridors. I became a little agitated and some of the nursing staff took notice.

Later that night, well past the time when visiting hours were over, I sat in my room with my good friends Hap and George. Hap and his wife Dan go way back with Laura and me. George had worked for me at two different dealerships. I hired him fresh out of Army recruiting. We developed a close friendship over the years; we share the same sense of humor! So, I was about as calm as I had been all day.

A knock on the door produced a tall bearded man, dressed in hospital garb and clasping a clipboard with files on it. That he was a doctor was immediately obvious to us all.

"Hi" he greeted us. "I hope I'm not interrupting anything but I was wondering if I could talk to you for a moment, Steve."

Hap and I had had a great visit, which I can clearly remember to this day. With a "Good luck buddy," he was gone. George, who had also done some work as a medic in the Army, could see it was time to leave and said good luck and goodbye. Dr. Berry sat down.

"I understand you are quite nervous about the procedure I am going to perform on you tomorrow, is that right?" he asked.

"How did you know that?" I replied, confirming his thoughts.

"Some of the nurses noticed that you seemed agitated and let me know. That is part of their job you see."

"Yeah, well, needles, especially like the one I guess you're gonna use tomorrow, are some of my least favorite things" I stated.

The good doctor went on to explain the procedure, predict what would be uncomfortable, how many thousands of times he has done it and its being done all over the world.

After this much needed talk and question answering session, he came to this rather impressive and absolute conclusion.

"I'll leave you with this thought Steve. You should be thrilled that I can perform this procedure on you, because, quite honestly, I would rather be shot than have the operation that angioplasty replaces!" This was an ominous statement, to say the least.

With that, he disappeared into the formless white corridors of the hospital, leaving me to my thoughts and worry. But I found that my worry was decreased a hundred fold. Just knowing exactly what would be on the agenda and who was going to do what helped calm me. After a short while I actually fell asleep.

My Heart Like A Roadmap

Five o'clock is not really early in the hospital. In fact, stuff goes on all night. When the nurses came in to wheel me out to the ambulance, I woke up and got with the program real quick. No breakfast, hit the head and let's go.

The ride in the ambulance was surreal. Thankfully, no siren but they ran the lights anyway.

"No, no, don't run the lights. I'm not gonna die or anything, just a routine procedure. Just drive like usual," I thought to myself. But we did make good time!

We went into the hospital, took a quick trip down an elevator and then into the room where they did angioplasty. They must have given me some relaxing drugs, because my heart should have been thumping. But I felt pretty calm. And I knew that I had to be almost fully awake for this procedure.

"Here we go," said doctor from the night before as he lifted my Johnny up and exposed my right thigh.

"I'm going to use this vein right here," he stated and indicated with a touch where he meant. "You might feel some discomfort for a brief moment as I get the catheter started, but it will be for just a moment."

He had touched me on my inner thigh about six inches down, and soon I felt the "discomfort." But true to his word, it subsided. Only later did I learn that the needle I felt was actually the Novocaine shot!

"I am now running the catheter up through your vein. Soon it will be stopped right in front of the main vein running into the heart," stated the doctor.

"OK, now I'm going to release a dye into your heart which will outline your arteries so we can locate and identify the blockages. They will show up on this monitor here right in front of you," he said. And for the first time since I had been lying there I noticed a monitor projected off to the side of my face. I could turn my head slightly and see it.

"OK, here we go," he said as he released the dye into my heart. "You may feel a little heat, you may feel flushed, it will just be momentary and is normal."

The dye was in. The monitor lit up with an image of my heart covered with red roads leading here and there.

"Is that my heart?" I rather stupidly blurted. But having never seen my heart like that, I didn't know what to say. It was beating and moving and I was looking at the monitor and feeling my heart at the same time!

"This is really bizarre," I thought to myself.

The mood in the room started to change. The doctor was printing something, a copy of what was being displayed on the monitor I guessed. He studied it, then said something about talking to his colleagues, and went over to another side of the room where I could see several other doctors gathered around. I lay there, looking at my heart and wondering if this guy would be able to fix it.

"I've got some bad news for you," he said glumly. "The blockages are too close, if I try to open one of the arteries, the other could burst, killing you right here on the table!"

This was the second time this week that a doctor had talked about me possibly dying! My spirit really started to drop! This was the same person who told me the night before that he would rather be shot than have the operation! And now he was telling me I would have the operation!

I freaked, panicked and then rallied, all at once.

"OK," I said. "Knock me out and do it right now!" I thought to myself this was a now or never thing. There was no way I was going to have the nerve to do this again.

"I'm sorry," he replied, smiling at my bravado. "The earliest we can operate is Monday morning." It was Friday morning at about seven am. Three long days loomed ahead of me like a dark gray cloud on my horizon!

I slumped back in my bed and started the procedure of internalizing everything that had just happened. After a moment of reflection I asked, "What's next?"

"A room is being prepared for you on the cardiac floor and you can just relax for a couple of days," he replied.

"Here we go again," I thought, "another room!"

Chapter Four

The Waiting Game, Part Two

The cardiac unit of CMC is the entire 4th floor. It is staggering at first to realize that all the patients on the floor are there for the same basic problem I was experiencing. Of course, I was the youngest that I could see, most patients being in their sixties or seventies. It didn't make me feel young, just out of place. The reality that people have their chests cut open and their hearts worked on by people who are like technicians repairing expensive equipment was impressive, but ominous.

My room was a double. My roommate was a very nice elderly gentleman named Al. Al was in his late seventies but seemed to have all his faculties, and we got to know each other as well as one does in the hospital. Because we were both scheduled for potentially life threatening surgery, a sort of camaraderie ensued. His family and mine talked about how they were coping with all this uncertainty, and they got along quite nicely.

The three days that were a lifetime crawled by. When the phone wasn't ringing and visitors weren't trying to entertain me, time seeped by, each moment becoming a chapter in the day. I could look out my window at the city of Manchester and see the daily hubbub. The feel of a weekend came through. This weekend would bring the end of life as I had known it; in fact that life was already gone. But Al and I kept each other's spirits up with false bravado and small talk. We kept it surface for the most part, neither one wanting to commit to a friendship that might not last the week.

Hey Doc, Would You Please Knock Me Out!

Five o'clock Monday morning finally came around. I thought of the irony that one week prior I had been up and getting ready to go to the gym for the beginning of yet another great day. But on this Monday, a redheaded nurse pushing a cart came strolling into the room. She exuded confidence and control and seemed nice enough.

Manchester has a large French-Canadian population, which is reflected in the staff of the hospital. As soon as she started to speak to me I could identify her French accent.

Annette was her name, and she parked the tray she was pushing next to my bed. Opening my Johnny, she soaped up my chest with a very strong astringent soap, and starting to shave what little blond chest hairs I am endowed with. Slapped in the face with the opening volley of what was to come, I observed,

"Ahhhh, this is kind of scary."

I don't know, maybe I was hoping she would stop, like my dentist when I move or grimace and groan, and wait for me to feel better about it. But she wasn't going to be deterred from performing her job.

"Now son," she purred, "you just lie back and relax, this is all out of your hands now, and in the hands of the good Lord!"

These words were meant to assure and placate me, but I was beginning to feel like I was being prepped for an execution, like all the bad movies I had seen in my life. I tried to keep the mind set that this was a huge effort being made to save and extend my life, that untold dollars would be spent this day on my behalf, and that grateful is how I should be feeling. But, unfortunately, my imagination was ruling the moment.

Finishing her duty, Annette packed up her tray and, like so many before her, flashed me a smile, wished me good luck, and melted away into the endless white corridors.

Soon another nurse entered the room. I was sure that similar events were happening to my roommate Al, but the curtains had been drawn and there was no communicating with my new friend. The nurse handed me two white pills and explained that they would relax me and make me sleepy. The anticipation was unreal.

A doctor and a team of orderlies arrived next. The curtains had been pulled back and Al was lying there looking just as apprehensive as me. Then, just as they were ready to wheel me out, there was some confusion. It seemed that Al would go first after all. No, Al had to go to another floor and have his carotids done first. So I would be first! "God, I hope they get it straight," I thought. But the Atavan was kicking in and I wasn't panicking.

The ride in the elevator to the Operating Room in the bowels of the hospital was as close to an out of body experience as I have ever known. The orderlies ignored me and their conversations seemed absolutely unreal. But the pills I was given, while producing an outstanding buzz, where not nearly

17

enough to knock me out. I'm not sure if it was because I was so wired, but I was really wide-awake.

The elevator door opened, and the lights from the OR shined out through the windows of the double doors in front of me. In a holding area outside the OR I was lined up with several other patients, who were destined for the same or similar fates as me. The orderlies, without so much as a goodbye or good luck, walked off, their conversation never missing a beat.

I lay there, wide-awake and thinking, "It just can't get any weirder than this!"

I noticed that the other patients were all out. I looked at them with envy, and wondered what was wrong with me.

Before abject panic could set in, a doctor dressed up like a scientist from NASA came strolling by, his hands held out in front of him, just like you see in the movies!

"Hey Doc," I said as he passed in front of me. "Would you please knock me out?"

He stopped abruptly, turned to me and asked, in a muffled voice through his mask, "Didn't they give you your pills?"

"Well, yeah, but I'm still wide-awake, see?" I said dragging my IV riddled arm off my chest to point at my eyes.

"I'll be right back," he assured me, moving off to a place I could not see. Soon he returned with a hypodermic needle and several small vials. As he drew some of the liquid out of each vial he explained,

"I'm mixing some narcotics that will knock you out, plus an amnesiac, you won't even remember this conversation!" he finished, as if he were apologizing for the pills not working.

At this point, I just wanted out. Knocked out. He placed the business end of the hypodermic in my IV and darkness flooded in on me. Strange, isn't it, that I remember that conversation?

Awake!

Consciousness was returning reluctantly, like a fourteen year old walking to the bus stop on Monday morning after a week's vacation.

I could hear voices, as if from a distance, one of them my wife I thought. My mouth and throat were parched. "Just swallow!" I was thinking. But that was not possible. I should be choking, but I wasn't. I opened my eyes. Oh, yeah, I remembered, the big one was upon me!

My wife and several other faces looked down at me. That in itself was a weird experience, because they were standing right over me. I wanted to speak, I always want to weigh in on any situation, but things seemed to be growing out of my mouth, tubes, a variety of tubes. I fell back to sleep. This was too much for my mind.

Some time later I felt the same sensations and I opened my eyes again. Things came into focus. There was a doctor futzing around doing doctor stuff. He looked over, and after what seemed a lifetime, noticed my open eyes.

"I think he's coming around this time," he observed.

I wanted to scream, "Yeah, I'm awake! Get this stuff out of my mouth!"

"Let's get these tubes out," he spoke to someone out of my sight, as if he could read my mind.

He grasped one of the tubes and started pulling it out of the desert that was my mouth. As the tube came out of my stomach, I sat up and started to gag. Gentle hands held me down. Moisture! The beginnings of relief! Then the other two tubes, one in each lung, came out.

"OK," I thought, "that's better." It was then I noticed my arm in a bandage, like it had been broken.

"Hmmmm, that's weird," was my response.

The drainage tubes jutting out of my chest were my next mental stop. "I'll just have to deal with that later." It was too much to try and take in all at once.

"You're back!" said the man who had been handling my heart for the last four or five hours.

"Water," I rasped back, like a soul lost for weeks on a shipwreck.

"Go easy," he said and put a straw to my lips.

The world was starting to come back into focus and with that the realization of what had just occurred to me. A level of comfort was returning. The worst was over.

"Take as big a breath as you can through this measuring device," the doctor requested as he handed me the clear plastic device. "We want to see how your lungs are doing."

The device he handed me was a clear plastic tube with a little ball sitting on the bottom of the tube. As you sucked in a breath, the ball floated up, and the measure of your breath intake was gauged by how far up the tube the ball was sucked.

I put the tube to my lips and breathed in as deeply as I could. It actually felt pretty good. The ball rose all the way to the top.

The doctor looked over, saw the ball at the top of the tube and said, "Can you do that again?"

"I'll try," I replied and repeated the performance.

"I'll be right back," he stated and disappeared. He returned with another doctor and two nurses.

"Can you repeat the breath test again?" He requested once more.

"OK." Once again the ball floated to the top of the tube.

Everyone looked at each other in amazement. "I've never seen that!" exclaimed the surgeon. "Never mind ICU, take him right to his room!"

Since that seemed to have gone so well, my native optimism started to blossom anew. I knew what had happened without an explanation having been given.

Weight bearing exercise has many excellent benefits, one of which is the expansion of lung capacity by using proper breathing techniques. And so, my many years of weight training had paid off in a rather large but unexpected way. I'm sure the many miles of running had been a major influence also.

I think it is important here to note that I lift weight for health and toning. It is kind of ironic that many people, mostly those who thought me crazy for my gym dedication, have said to me, "Aren't you mad now that you spent all that time at the gym. You had a heart attack anyway!"

A year or so after the dust had settled I was visiting my doctor for my regular six-month checkup. The nurse who was prepping me had some interesting information. We were having a discussion about the nature and type of my "event" and I mentioned that the doctor had said I might not survive the attack. Looking at my records, she agreed that the survival rate for the magnitude of the cardiac arrest I experienced was not good. I mentioned my workout routine and asked if she thought it had any bearing on my survival. She explained to me that when someone challenges their heart regularly, with weight bearing exercise and regular cardio workouts, that the heart actually grows many little capillary veins, the small veins that are the last line in the blood distribution network. These extra little capillary veins were able to supply my heart with enough blood to keep my heart alive until the clot busting drugs could do their jobs!

I knew that my exercise had many benefits. After that discussion, my observations were justified and I had a good reply to my skeptics!

"No, I don't regret one single moment of working out. If I hadn't done it I would be dead now!" became my answer. And that really does say it all!

My Room

The attendant brought me to my room. It was not the same one I had been in. That was a bit of a surprise. I had been looking forward to seeing my pal Al. I was anxious to compare notes and see how he had made out. A man a little older than me occupied the new room. He was a large man. You could tell that even though he was in bed. He seemed to nod slightly to me as I was wheeled by. The curtain was pulled for privacy and soon I was back to sleep. My main objective now was to sleep, heal, and recover.

After a short period of sleeping, I was awakened by a lot of rather loud talking and laughter coming from the other side of the curtain. I waited, hoping the people would remember I was on the other side and might want to sleep. NO dice, the noise got louder and louder. I rang for the nurse.

"Could you ask the folks next door to quiet down a little, I really just want to sleep," I requested of the nurse. She agreed that the noise level was annoying.

After a quick trip to the other side of the room, she returned with an aggravated look on her face.

"These folks are not very nice and they said you just have to put up with their noise, they think they are entitled and that's that!" She informed me.

I thought to myself that these were not my kind of people, and rolled over to try to sleep. As it turned out, he was getting ready to be discharged, so I decided to just wait it out.

Later that afternoon, just as he was about to leave, he came over to my side of the curtain, looking to see if I was awake.

"How you feeling?" he seemed to genuinely inquire.

"Tired but OK," was my reply.

The number of IVs and other apparatus that were protruding from all parts of my body were abundant. One of these items was a small wire jutting out of my chest right where my heart would be, partially covered by a band-aid. Mr. Jolly pointed to this and asked, "Do you know what that is for?"

I looked where he was pointing and admitted I did not.

"That little wire goes directly into your heart, it's there in case you start to flat line, they can jump-start you with it!" He seemed delighted to inform me.

"OK," I thought. "It seems reasonable that they would take some precautions".

"Yeah," he continued. "The last thing they do before you can go home is to pull that right out!"

"OK," I once again thought, "that makes sense."

"Boy, does that hurt," he continued. I was starting to figure out where this dude was coming from.

"When they pulled mine out, I could feel it coming right out of my heart!" he went on. "And when it was out, I saw the doctor looking at the piece of meat that came out, stuck on the end of the wire where it was attached to my heart!"

"Thanks," was all I said, sarcastically.

With that, he seemed satisfied enough to say "See Ya!" and was gone, leaving me with the dread that I'm sure he knew would result from his tale. That I have never seen him again suits me swell!

CHAPTER FIVE

Getting Up

My procedure had included a double bypass, and once again, my weight training had paid off. Instead of using veins from my legs, as is common, an artery in my arm was used. That explained the cast-like bandage on my left arm. The benefits of using an artery are two fold. The first is that the removal of veins from the legs can cause a painful recovery. And I was determined to get back to running! The second is that arteries are used in the blood system to take blood away from the heart while veins are the return pipes. The net result is that an artery will last longer as a graft.

The same day that they rewire your heart, they expect you to get up and sit in a chair. I was sure they were kidding, but they were serious. So later that same day, two nurses came in. Their goal was to get me into a chair. The many tubes, wires and IVs complicated the simple feat of getting up.

With the help of my two nurses, I was soon sitting in a comfortable chair next to my bed. Laura was sitting on the bed looking at me, and I remember her saying she couldn't believe I was sitting on a chair the same day my heart had been operated on. But there I was, drainage tubes coming out of my chest and emptying into a plastic container, IVs sprouting from all parts of my body like weeds, and a urinary catheter slithering menacingly out from under my johnny! I was wondering how I was going to get back in the bed now that I was out!

I was back in bed a little while later. The nurses have a system that seemed to work like a well-oiled machine.

I wanted to know when I could go home. Afraid that I might be laughed at, I was surprised at the serious look on the RN's face when she said, "You will be home by the weekend!"

It seemed unbelievable that they could open me, bypass my heart with a machine to keep me alive while they rewired me, plug my heart back in, sew me up and in four days send me home!

As it turned out, I was to be discharged on Thanksgiving Day!

Thanksgiving is a big event for my family. We usually have around thirty people and rent a big hall to accommodate everyone. Relatives come from Massachusetts and Connecticut, so they all stay overnight. It's a real old-fashioned Thanksgiving! I would miss this one, but there should be more to come!

However, I had a job to do before Thanksgiving. The nurses were great, so encouraging and friendly. But they had rules. One of the rules was you couldn't go home if you didn't eat, and then process that food through the final act of voiding. This doesn't seem like a big deal, but after what I had gone through it actually was.

Hospital food is not so bad, but after major heart surgery, nothing really looked appetizing. Picking three meals a day from the daily menu doesn't sound hard to do, but when the thought of food is less than appealing, it is the hardest part of the day.

When the food was delivered, the real work began. I would try to eat enough that the nurses would take the tray away without those disapproving looks. The little that I did eat did not allow me to achieve the goal set for me.

The Wednesday before Thanksgiving Day, my wife and I were treated to a visit from two old friends of ours. Bob and Pam had been friends for twenty years or more and had made the effort to see me in the hospital. I later found out that the number of people who had had come to see me was substantial. My memory at best is spotty, and being focused on getting out, some visits were forgotten. But Bob and Pam's had an even more desirable effect than just some support and well wishing.

Pam is the producer of tollhouse cookies that look, smell and taste like manna from heaven. She had come that day armed to the teeth with a plate of her special fare. My first reaction was sadness that I wouldn't be enjoying them. I had no interest in them and I was sure they were way off any diet that a person just out of heart surgery should have. I thought it best that I share them with those who would enjoy them.

As the nurses came in, I would offer them each a cookie. After some cajoling, each would accept and if they ate it right then, the "oooooooos" and "ahhhhhhhs" as Pam's tollhouse cookies hit home were substantial.

Later that night the head nurse came in and suggested I try one of those thick, chocolate chip riddled cookies before they were all gone. I protested for a bit, and then finally, to appease her, I picked one up and took a bite. Chocolate chips filled my mouth, offset by sweet tollhouse cookie dough.

24

My stomach instantly sat up and took notice. "More of that!" came the order from my stomach. I was off and ready to eat!

The cookies had done their job, my appetite was back, and the end result of a perfectly formed stool made my exit a sure thing.

Thanksgiving morning, Thursday of the same week as my surgery, I was ready to go home!

Ready To Go Home

When Thursday morning arrived Laura and I were given some discouraging news.

"Yes, you are ready to go home, but the discharge nurse won't be in today," the nurse in charge told us.

I'm always hard pressed to take no for an answer, but this day was really going to test me.

"There must be someone else who can cut me out of here," I stated.

Laura could see I was ready to go and knew that nothing short of getting out would satisfy me. She was in charge of thirty guests and wouldn't mind me staying in the hospital and out of her way for another day. I was adamant, I wanted out. And after all that had happened to me, I didn't think it unreasonable to want to be placated.

Finally, Laura and the nurse agreed that I should be discharged. The discharge person was contacted and asked if she would accommodate me. And she did!

The last thing, of course, that had to be done was remove all of the tubes, IVs' and wires from my body. I began to get apprehensive. I couldn't help but remember my unpleasant roommate and his tale of pain and anguish when the wire in his heart was removed.

"The doctor will be in soon to remove your tubes and wires," my nurse informed me. I began to sweat. For the next two hours I sat there and soon the sweat was literally pouring out of my head. I went through an entire box of tissue.

Finally, the doctor came into my room to pull my tubes. He greeted me jovially and spoke about me going home and how great that was. Then he held my tubes firmly in his hands and asked if I was ready. As I was saying "yes" he pulled and the two tubes came out of my chest rather painlessly.

"OK, that was done," I thought. "Now for the rest of the stuff!"

The nurse was taking out IVs. As she removed the one from my neck she explained that it went all the way to my heart. It was to provide a chemical path for stimulants in case my heart had stopped! Out it came, without difficulty. Before I knew it, the wire from my chest was gone also. My mean-hearted roommate had needlessly caused a lot of worry and anxiety.

Graduation Day

One of the things that had perplexed me was there was no sign of my old roommate Al. When I would inquire about him, everyone just said they didn't know, and when pressed they said things like "he must have been transferred" or some other excuse.

When the discharge nurse had given me her regular speech and instructions, I was ready to go. The last thing Laura and I wanted was to know about Al. Laura knew I would like to say goodbye and wish him luck. She called the front desk to ask if he was still registered with the hospital. The discharge nurse had a strange look on her face as she overheard Laura's phone conversation.

Laura hung up and said to me, "They don't have anyone by that name registered here!"

We thought that was strange, and were looking at each other uncomfortably, when the nurse finally said, "There is a reason he's not registered. Your roommate didn't make it through the operation."

Laura and I sat in stunned silence for a moment.

"Wow!" was all I could muster.

"We didn't want to tell you about it for fear that it would upset you," she explained.

"I have been more upset by the pussyfooting around and confusion!" I replied. I was frustrated but I felt a little foolish. I knew deep down that they had been trying to prevent me from becoming upset.

After some talk and further inquiries about the family, I decided to move on and focus on the job at hand, getting home.

The discharge process over, I started to get up to head for the door.

"Not so fast!" said one of the nurses still hovering around me. I thought that after being in their care they were finding it hard to cut the ties! In reality, they wanted me to wait for the wheelchair that was going to be my transportation to the front door.

"I can walk!" I exclaimed. I was thinking this was the start of my recovery. But this was another rule the hospital wouldn't bend. Because of liability, if you want to walk out the front door, fine, but they will get you there in a wheelchair.

At the front door, things started to get a little emotional for me. The whole experience seemed to amplify my emotions.

Between the drugs and the emotional highs and lows, a good cry was never very far away. The good-byes at the hospital door were more emotional than I had expected. I felt like I had graduated from some unbelievable academy where I had done well and now could go out into the world.

With a final wave, Laura started the car and headed for the pharmacy. The new life I would begin would include drugs. Several such drugs, designed to prevent a repeat experience, were soon a part of my daily regimen.

There was a beta-blocker for my heart rate, Zocor for my cholesterol, and Percocet for pain. Don't forget an aspirin a day!

With bags full of drugs, we headed home.

Home Sweet Home

Words can't describe how beautiful my humble home looked to me after several weeks away.

Laura took my arm and slowly we went up the steps to the front door, trying not to get the old heart rate up too much! I walked in the door and I was home!

I stood there looking around and letting my familiar surroundings soak in. It was then that it hit me, not only was I still alive, I was home. And home is where they love you!

I looked out my window at the lake; it would be frozen over soon. The air was chilly, and yet crisp and clean after the smells of the hospital.

It was Thanksgiving. I felt, and I know my family felt, that we all had something to be really thankful for. Of course, I would not be able to go across the lake to the big hall we rent for our festivities, but just knowing that everyone was there and I was home was great!

Over the course of the next two days, friends and family from our Thanksgiving party came to visit me in ones and twos. They were extremely considerate, and tried not to overstay and tire me out. I was so moved to see everyone that I didn't show them how exhausted I really was.

Tears Of Joy

When my heart attack occurred, we all agreed that it would do no good to tell my mother about it. We made up a story about pneumonia, and that seemed to satisfy her curiosity. Telling her would only create more stress and worry for her given our family history of heart disease, herself included. Adjusting to the recent experience of living in a nursing home was difficult enough we decided

My mother had lived with us for five years. She was able to get to know my two kids while being part of the family, and was a huge contribution to the household.

We had sold the home in Massachusetts that she and my Dad had bought in 1954. We built Mom a first-floor apartment in our house. She had her own entry, car, bathroom, dining area and living room. She had brought all her own furniture with her, and when she would head downstairs we kidded her that she was headed for Wakefield, the town in Massachusetts where she had lived all her life.

So for five great years we all lived together, helping and nurturing each other and making a happy home. Fortunately, she was with us the night she suffered her heart attack. She was taking dinner, as she did each night, with my wife and two children. I was working. Laura noticed my Mom not looking right and began questioning her.

Laura determined Mom was having a heart attack and wanted to call an ambulance. Mom would have none of that, insisted on putting on some makeup and said, "Laura would you please drive me to St. Joe's!"

Mom returned home after a brief stay and a double angioplasty performed by the same doctor who did my angiogram.

She enjoyed another year or two of good health, and then the aging process took its toll.

All good things must end, and Mom reached the point where she needed more help than we could provide. So, reluctantly, she moved into a nursing home fifteen minutes from me. Laura had done a lot of comparisons, and we found it an extremely clean and well-organized facility. I would drop in to see her frequently as my work took me in that general direction. Also, my favorite billiards parlor was around the corner! The nurses never knew when I would show up, morning, lunch or dinner!

When I arrived home, I wanted desperately to see her. But I could not go out, and she could not physically come into my house. It would take a wheelchair and several assistants to accomplish this. So, my sister Holly drove Mom to my house where I could wave out the window to her. I made a large sign that said, "I love you, MOM!" I held it up to the window so she could see. I was crying, she was crying, and Holly was crying. But, I did get to see her and let her know I loved her. It was as good as it was going to get for a while, and it was pretty good.

And so I was home, Thanksgiving came and went, along with all our family and friends, and my recovery was in full swing!

CHAPTER SIX

Walking With Julie

My existence became an exercise in trying to regain my life. My first shower was an experience that stands out vividly in my mind. I had a fresh wound on my chest and arm and the first time I exposed it to the rushing water was nerve racking.

When the surgeons had finished with me, the only trace of entry into my chest was a very fine line going down my middle from the sternum to just above my naval. It was one of the wonders of the operation! My visitors were treated to this sight at the merest request, sometimes a request I may have almost prompted. Because, this was a real work of art! A regular Rembrandt! In fact, had the truth been known, I was proud of this scar.

The wound on my arm ran from the crook of my elbow to about an inch from my wrist. This wound had stitches on it. The chest incision had been closed with sutures that are inside and just deteriorate away.

The net result was an intense feeling of vulnerability.

With some help from Laura, I got in and out of the shower OK. This small act helped jump-start my mental recovery. Because, now I knew that some things would return to normal.

On day two I started the walking routine that my doctors had outlined. I was to go to the end of the street and back, not too fast. I had to give the grafts time to heal and I didn't want to rush things and end up back where I started.

My daughter Julie, who was eight years old at this time, wanted to walk with me. I'll never forget the first time. It was a cold day, but sunny. We dressed warmly, and holding her little hand in mine we went forth. She would go with me each day after that. She would hold my hand and out the door we would go.

I was so inspired by being home, and assisted in my daily walks by my little girl, that I could see myself returning to the gym. Before I went back, however, I felt as though I should thank the people there because if it hadn't been for them I wouldn't be here. So, inspired, I sat down and penned a letter to the editor of our local newspaper. This is what I wrote:

Nashua Telegraph
December 9, 1998

Gold's Gym Staff Saw Fatal Signs

To the Editor:

Several weeks ago, after finishing a routine workout at Gold's Gym in Nashua, I began feeling not quite right, somehow different. Since I work out regularly and have for some years, a heart attack was not something I was suspicious of.

However, the professional trainers at Gold's Gym picked up on my apparent uneasiness and quite literally saved my life! A heart attack, quite severe, was, in fact, exactly what was happening.

Thanks to Chris, Craig and Abdel for recognizing the symptoms of cardiac arrest and forcing me to believe it!

Special thanks to my friend Abdel, for knowing when to hit the mule on the head with a two by four! And club member Joe Yanco, for calmly calling my wife to notify her. Rockingham Ambulance Service and emergency room personnel at St. Joseph Hospital in Nashua, where Dr. Liebling saved my life much in the same manner saved my mother's life six years ago!

After an angiogram and double bypass surgery at Catholic Medical Center in Manchester, I am now on my way to a full recovery.

The outpouring of concern and consideration I have experienced in these past weeks has been truly moving and undoubtedly helped my recovery. It will be a while until I'm recovered enough to return to Gold's Gym, but all I can say is, "I'll be back!"

Steve Jaynes Sr.
Merrimack

Just putting these words down on paper made me feel better, and when the letter was published and I saw it in print; I started to believe it myself!

For the next week, Julie walked with me almost every day. I got stronger and stronger. Then, I started to feel like I was losing ground.

When Staff Turns Inward

Ten days after being discharged from CMC, I really started to feel poorly. My hips ached, and walking was hard.

That night I got up in the middle of the night to relieve myself, and looking down I saw puss leaking out of the base of my incision. All the good things in my life began swirling down a vortex, which lead directly to hell. I knew one thing instantly. My world was crumbling once again!

We live in a world of germs and bacteria, viruses and their numerous mutations. And a very simple and common bacterium is called staphylococcus.aureus. These bacteria are all around us, on us and in the air. Almost always, they are harmless and no doubt play an important roll in the chain of life that makes up our universe.

Doctors don't know why, when or necessarily how these bacteria decide to become anaerobic and turn inside a host.

I've never been accused of being the perfect host, but at some point either during the operation or after, one or some of these little bastards got into the wound in my chest. There they lived very happily, eating my flesh and swimming in my blood. Conditions inside me were so lovely for these nasty creatures that they multiplied like, well, bacteria.

By the time they decided to make their presence known by making an exit and flowing down my belly, the reproduction of their clan put my sedentary blood count just before the point when they pronounce you dead.

Ten days after my glorious departure I arrived at CMC feeling like dead weight. This time when they greeted me with a wheelchair at the door, I gladly accepted.

I was whisked away to the office of the doctor that had performed my double bypass. I seemed to have gotten a magic pass. No waiting, go right in Mr. Jaynes! They rushed me into his office and then right into an exam room.

There was not a lot of talk at first. I was given the old line, "We have to see what we're dealing with." I knew what we were dealing with. I was infected!

Without any warning or talk, the doctor took up a large swab stick and started towards the little hole the pus was seeping out. I wasn't thinking anything particularly horrible was about to happen when he jammed the entire end of the swab into the hole! He then gave it a few little twists. If I hadn't known he was an actual doctor I would have mistaken him for a torture expert!

Leaving the swab sticking out of my belly, he turned away from me. Finally he turned back and, giving the stick one more twist, removed the swab. After a brief inspection, he stuffed it into a tube.

"Whatcha gonna do with that?" I inquired, feeling that since it had been forcibly removed from my body I had the right to know.

"Send it out to research to find out exactly what kind of bug we are working with here," was the reply.

"Oh yeah," I was thinking. "Bugs, probably millions, living in my chest and eating me alive!"

I started to have another of out of body experience, and it was getting ugly. I hovered above the bed, one eye on the proceeding, the other looking for the fastest way out if it became necessary. I watched in horror and amazement as my surgeon of the week before, my hero who hath bestowed life back upon me, took a hypodermic needle and drew some Novocaine into it.

"What's up with that, doc?" I said, wishing I hadn't because I really didn't want to hear the answer.

"Just a little Novocaine, I need to see what's going on here," he replied, like he was making me buttered toast.

With mounting terror, I watched my savior pick up a nasty looking knife and turn to my stomach, just above my naval. He was looking at the spot where the pus was still flowing. With several quick strokes, he cut out a chunk of meat about the size of a quarter, deep enough to put a marble in. The crevice instantly started to pool up with blood and pus.

The real me knew that this was happening to someone who just looked like me, that no such thing would ever happen in real life. The guy on the table, the guy with the hole in his stomach that was overflowing with lots of blood and pus now, he was really starting to get sick.

I'm not one to be lost for words. It's kind of a joke with my friends and family. But I had nothing to say. I was in shock. I guess it must be how victims feel.

The two doctors left. Before they did, one put a gauze pad over my new wound, which was starting to overflow and run down my stomach.

One In A Hundred Club

As the doctors made their exit, my wife was let in to see me. She saw the gauze pad on my belly and just sort of looked at me. I could see the panic building up in her eyes as she started coming to the same unconfirmed conclusions that I had.

Laura comforted me as best she could, but the sensation of the world spinning out of control was getting stronger now. One thing that was just a harbinger of things to come was, no pain meds. Painkillers were handed out meagerly at best, and I came to call these guys the "bring your own dope" doctors.

After a while, the doctors came back in. They were part of a team of professionals; they had their own company and were reputed to be among the best in world. CMC has very progressive, state of the art, trend setting Cardio-thoracic department. These guys are considered pioneers!

The doctors looked at my wife and I, and I could see real concern for us. That was probably the scariest look that has ever been cast my way.

"Your husband has an infection, probably staff, but we are waiting to confirm the exact type that has gotten into him. We do know that it is a bacterium. Steve is going to have to be admitted and will need debreeding. The nurses are taking care of his admitting right now."

I didn't know what debreeding meant but I was pretty sure I could live without knowing. The guy hovering over me knew I was going to find out. There was no place to escape to; my reality had become a feeling of panic and fear.

In an effort to make me feel better, or more likely to make himself feel better, one of the doctors slapped my good arm and said, "Well, you are one in one hundred!"

He explained that CMC has a one percent infection rate, while the rest of the country averages three percent. I was their one in one hundred.

Feelings of anger began to crop up. I knew instinctively that this would take off like a California forest fire if not checked. I started taking slow breaths and tried to come to terms with my bad luck. I decided that I absolutely had to let the anger go. It would consume me, and put my wife over the edge. So I acted like that was great news, and the guy hovering over me was a little surprised.

After a few more moments of discussion, the nurse came in and helped me into the wheelchair. Up a corridor to the elevator and right to the cardiac floor, floor four.

I looked for familiar faces and saw some. Everyone was busy with their various assignments, but some smiled pathetically at me while others just kind of shook their heads in some kind of display of mutual sadness at my return. When you come back to cardio, and it's not cardio rehab, it ain't good!

This time I had my own private room. Later I discovered that it is almost always reserved for the one in a hundred winners - like myself. This is to keep the germs localized in one room and to isolate infected patients.

I Learn A New Word

After I was resituated in my new room and had received some drugs and comfort, the doctor representing the surgery team came to my room.

"We have diagnosed the bacteria as staff, a certain type which we know how to fight. That is the good news," he offered in an official voice meant to relay confidence and wisdom.

"Steve will have to be opened up. The infection is all through his chest, and he will need debreeding." This was the second time I heard that word. I had to ask what it meant.

"Doc, exactly what do you mean by debreeding?" I asked, hoping the guy still hovering over me was the real me so I could get the answer, wish the poor bastard lying on the bed good luck, and head home.

"We must go into your wound and remove everything that has been contaminated by the bacteria," he stated, obviously holding back the more graphic details he could have provided. My overworked imagination was having a field day with that stuff anyway, I doubt if he could have come up with anything worse than what I was thinking.

"So, when does this debreeding begin?" I asked.

"We have an operating room scheduled for tomorrow morning, so get as much rest as you can tonight," he replied.

With that the doctor left, and Laura and I were left alone for the first time to look at each other and try to size up our lot. In typical fashion, her first words were "I'm sorry, honey."

Like this could be her fault! I had no reply. I didn't even chastise her, as I'm apt to do for her apologizing for something that she didn't cause. All I could do was lay there, feeling horrible, and wonder how my life could be returned to me only to be snatched away again!

After some talk, hugging, and optimistic phrases, Laura headed home to see to the house and kids. There were bills to still be paid, time marched on!

The calendar had just turned to December, a time of hope and fun and gifts and presents. I knew the work and planning that went into these celebrations and the thought needed to effectively buy gifts for kids. These concerns were on my mind as I lay there looking at Laura, and through her eyes, our children.

"Go home and tell the kids it is going to be all right," I told her. She agreed that the kids needed her more than me and finally tore herself away from the special room where the one in a hundred stay and headed home.

Doc, Make Me A Promise!

Later that afternoon towards dinner time, the anesthesiologist who would be in charge of my lack of consciousness came to visit me. He appeared in my room quietly. He was a quiet spoken man, and seemingly compassionate.

After answering his questions about allergic reactions, weight and other things that concern such experts, it occurred to me that he was also responsible for the urinary catheter that I so unpleasantly awoke with from my initial operation. Of all the tubes and wires I had had removed or stuck in me, the catheter from my prize possession was ultimately horrifying and unpleasant. Anticipation of another experience like that was starting to overtake my general horror. I was starting to panic and look for a quick way out.

"So doc," I began carefully, not knowing exactly how to get into this with him, "are you also in charge of the urine catheter?"

"Yes, that is one of my responsibilities," he relied professionally.

"Boy, I really hate them," I offered.

"A little discomfort but they serve their purpose and help you to recover from these severe operations," he rationalized.

"Yeah, but doc, I really hate those things," I repeated. This time I could see a little concern in his eyes.

"The discomfort is small in comparison to the benefit of not having to get up to urinate. It allows the wound to heal without being disturbed," he continued, regaling me with looks of understanding and sorrow at the need to cause me this "discomfort."

"Look, doc," I began, "I can very easily urinate into a container while lying in bed if you are concerned about me getting up, but I really don't want another catheter".

"I'm sorry, but the operation is going to be pretty long and you absolutely need to be catheterized for it. Sorry," he finished.

But I was not done. Years of selling and dealing with hard ass managers had taught me to persevere when I felt correct; I gently pressed on,

"So, how about you do what you have to and, just before I wake up, you remove the catheter?" I offered and requested at the same time.

He thought about that for a minute in silence, then asked,

"You think you can urinate into a container while in bed?" He mused aloud. "I guess that would work OK, plenty of patients do that when they have to."

"Doc, I've been through a lot and this would mean a lot to me if you would help me out with this," I continued in my best closing voice.

Looking now for a commitment, I finished with, "So please promise me that you won't forget or let the other doctors talk you out of this, promise me I won't wake up with a plastic tube stuck in my dick!"

Guys, even doctors, like to talk trash once in while, so I mixed some humor in with my close and, with a laugh and a handshake, we agreed, no catheter when I woke up.

Convincing the doctor to remove the unpleasant tube before I woke up was nothing less than a single victory; I was feeling a little bit in charge of myself again, at last!

The day came to a close, and the nights that aren't really nights in the hospital began. I tried to sleep, and the guy hovering over me slowly descended and we became one

CHAPTER SEVEN

Have Your Seen Your Wound

As the little edges of reality started to poke at my awareness, sensations of being hit by a truck became more intrusive. I struggled to remain in the world of the unconscious. This was the place I wanted to stay, because no recent experience in reality seemed nearly as peaceful.

I can still remember the voices, quietly spoken as though in a library. My eyes were still closed, but slowly opening. I looked around, and my first thought was to feel for the dreaded catheter. True to his word, the good doctor had removed it.

Soon, the recovery room nurse came to inquire of my comfort. After a while, since there seemed no more point in keeping me in recovery, they took me to my private room.

There was a large bandage covering my chest, I could tell that even though the blanket was pulled up to my neck. The bandage felt really strange, kind of loose if that makes any sense.

We arrived in my room and the nurse busied herself with her chores. This was different from the return to my room after my bypass. This event was unfortunate, something bad had happened. Even though a heart attack is traumatic, the knowledge that the next operation is designed to get you back to normal, that the future is bright, makes the mood optimistic.

The mood now was quiet, let the poor man sleep, the unfortunate bastard! Imagine going through all that just to have it all removed; all the stitches, all the wires holding my chest together, and of course, all the infected flesh and bone.

As the day wore on, it became apparent that the routine here was going to be quite different from the previous one. Instead of, "hey let's get up today." it was, in a quiet sad kind of voice, "it's time to change your dressing."

A dreaded voice said just that, "Time to change your dressing." then, "Have you seen your wound yet?"

The voice belonged to a nice, rather young and pretty nurse who obviously knew what she was doing as she prepared some articles next to my bed and started turning down the bed sheet.

The last time I had seen my "wound", it looked as I described earlier, like a single red line running down my chest to my stomach, a quintessential zipper. It was the kind of scar people joke about. "Hey, you're a member of the zipper club!" you might hear with a guffaw. I was even oddly proud of my scar, so I was not really prepared for the new, improved wound.

A crevice several inches across, and deep enough to reveal lungs and ribs, stretched from the top of my chest all the way down to just above my naval. It was filled with cotton baton soaked in diluted bleach. And I was to discover that for the next several weeks, twice a day those bleach soaked cotton pads would have to be replaced.

The true meaning of the word "debreeding" had finally been revealed to me.

I wish I could have remained ignorant.

My Higher Power

The next two weeks were hell. At one point I lost the will to live. Between being sick from the infection, weakened by the latest operation and the twice-daily routine of changing the cotton, I was mentally beat.

A nurse would come in to my room one hour before it was time to change the cotton. I would get one or two Atavan, a real strong drug that makes you feel like it would be OK to tear an arm or two off.

In addition to the Atavan, I had my own morphine pump. I could press the button every seven minutes and receive a new dose of morphine.

So when the nurses gave me the Atavan, I knew what was coming. I would watch the clock, stare at the clock and every seven minutes on the nose, click the button for more dope in order to prepare myself for the debreeding.

The pain was so unreal. The baring of my vital organs twice a day was so mentally pummeling, no matter how many times I hit the morphine, no matter how many Atavan they gave me, it was unbearable. It was like having my chest torn open twice a day.

After a few days the nurses started to hear my negative talk, and they became concerned. I told them not to worry, I was a come from behind, rally kind of guy. In reality though, I was beat. I was ready to throw in the proverbial towel.

One day, after almost two weeks of this routine, I had just plain had it! The nurse came in with my atavan to announce the one-hour countdown to the bandage nurse. I should prepare myself. This was the second time that day, and it was just too much.

"Tell her not to bother, I quit," I said.

"What do you mean, you quit?" came the question.

"I'm done, I can't do this anymore," I whined.

"Sure you can," came the expected reply.

I wasn't ready for what followed.

"God never gives you more that you can handle," she offered.

To myself I thought "standard religious bullshit," but to her I said, "Well, he's given me more than I can handle."

"Have you asked him for help?" she continued.

"No, I'm not a religious person," I explained.

"Well, I'm going to close the door and leave you in privacy for a while. People pray to God however they are moved. Ask God for help and he will give you some strength."

With that she gathered up her items and, with a smile that said, "I mean it!" she left. She left me alone with my pain, my thoughts and my despair.

I thought about what she had said, and compared that to my own beliefs concerning God, life and the energy force from which we must all be created. And I started to pray. I prayed to God, to my higher power, Jesus, Allah, any name I could think of. I closed my eyes and actually started to cry. Tears of frustration, anger that this could happen to me, loneliness. There is nothing as lonely as a hospital room.

Time stood still, that was not unusual in my room. But as I prayed and asked for strength, a feeling of calmness descended over me. I'm sure a Christian would say the Holy Spirit was in me. I guess a Muslim would say Allah had touched me. I don't claim to know, I asked for help from just plain God. My God. Not the God of a church. Not some sacred ritual performed by costumed men or women. It was just me, in the privacy of my room, asking for help in the form of the will to live, to get through this hell.

And so I received help from God, and I have never felt the need to classify, categorize or otherwise explain the phenomenon. I am grateful, and try to remember to be every day. I believe that if people are in need of help from God, we are able to tap into that energy force by focus, and prayer can be a form of focus.

But I digress, and this is not a book about how to find God. Maybe I'll write that another time! I'm not so sure God didn't find me!

Finally, the door opened and a nurse with the tray of new cotton entered, somewhat hesitantly. She must have heard of my attitude of surrender. But I displayed none of that. I winced slightly as she tore the bandage open. The tape tore more skin off my chest, which already was a patchwork of torn tape marks. As she pulled the old cotton from my wound and inspected the area, she asked how I was doing.

"I'm OK," was all I felt I needed to reply. The feeling of calm remained, and I knew I could do this.

"How's it look?" I asked.

"Actually, I'm starting to see some new growth were they debreeded you. That's a good sign!" she finished.

I wanted to tell the nurse who had convinced me to ask for help thanks, that her advice had been perfect. I sometimes wonder if she had any idea how powerful her words were. My instinct tells me that she has given that very advice many times before, and since. I hope her words help her other charges like they did me. Because, right then and there the whole terrible ordeal started to turn around!

Danny's Little Friend

One afternoon I was lying in bed thinking positive thoughts to keep my spirits up. My window looked out at the Manchester airport and I could always see, day or night, a constant stream of planes flying in and out of the city.

Across a parking lot was another building, another part of the hospital. That afternoon, as I looked out hoping for something interesting to watch, a small bird came zooming down out of the sky and actually landed on the side of the other building! Upon closer inspection, I discovered it was one of the peregrine falcons that had come to make the city their home. There were several nest sites known and a camera had been set up to view one of them. So this was a treat, I love nature stuff.

I heard a slight knock on the door, and looked over to see my good friend Danny standing just inside, looking for approval to enter. For Danny to knock on my door was unnecessary, he was welcome anytime. And in fact he had spent a fair amount of time visiting with me, often after visiting hours had ended. As a member of the one in a hundred club, the rules got bent easily.

We all have friends, some we consider to be close, and others who are really acquaintances. So many of my good friends came and supported me while I was sick. The majority of those visits, I'm sorry to say, have been forgotten; not so much forgotten as not remembered. I like to think the morphine had a lot to do with that. The doctors mentioned several times the amnesiac properties of today's drugs. This visit of Danny's I remember.

My friendship with Danny went back to my early days at the gym. I had joined D.R. Fitness, a little hole in the wall, to get out of the rain and snow when I wanted to run and the weather was "NewEnglanding." Ninety-nine dollars a year and I could have a treadmill anytime I wanted. But Doug, the owner, after watching me come in and run for several months, approached me and encouraged me to do some cross training.

"It will improve your running!" he baited me. God knew my running could use improvement!

So cross training became part of my regimen, and after a while I got to know some of the people in the gym. Not that I wanted to. I met people all day in my position then as sales manager for a medium sized Chrysler franchise. A quick workout and on my way was my goal.

But I am a social guy, and after a while I knew all the characters. Many of them eventually bought cars and trucks from me.

But there was this one dude, skinny and kind of quiet, who came in, got on the stepper, worked up a good sweat for an hour, and then would leave. There was something about his looks that I didn't like. And I made up my mind that he would not be someone I could like.

One day this fella gets off the stepper he had been using, dries off and comes over to me where I was training with a bench press.

Sticking out his hand to me, he said, "Hi, my name is Danny, and I noticed that you talk to everyone in the gym but me. Can I be your friend too?"

I was floored, and instantly embarrassed! Was I being that obvious that I thought bad thoughts about him?

"Oh yeah, of course," was my weak reply.

As the weeks went by, Danny and I would occasionally work out together. It turned out that he was also a salesman, and the things we had in common became more and more obvious as our friendship developed.

To this day, I don't know what Danny saw in me that he would go to that much trouble to get to know me, but I sure am glad he did. His family and mine are very close and Danny is the best friend you could ever have.

This day, Danny, who walks with a good-natured bounce like JA JA Binks in the Star Wars movie, had a young boy with him. Danny had two boys of his own then but this little boy was a new face to me.

"Hey, Danny, what's up? Who you got with ya?" I asked.

"I want you to meet my little friend Tony."

Tony held out a small hand and shook mine gently, like he was a full-grown man trying not to be too forceful.

"Hi Tony, thanks for coming to see me," I said, not sure why he was here but happy to see such a promising young face with a radiant smile.

After some lighthearted banter and back and forth news, Danny said Tony had something he wanted to say to me. Then, Tony started to tell his story.

It seems that this boy had been born with half a heart! He had already had three operations, all more serious and severe than mine, and was facing the prospect of several more as he grew up. As he told his tale and we shared some mutual experiences, it became clear to me why Danny had brought this young boy to me. Get on with it, was the message. Hurry up and get better, there is basketball to play and pizza that needs eating! We aren't going to let a little heart problem stop us from that, are we?

Tony finished his little motivational piece by urging me, "C'mon, Steve, if I can do it, so can you!"

"Thanks, thanks so much Tony for sharing this with me," was the best I could do.

"Before I go, I want to give you this," the eight year old said. Digging into his child size jeans pocket, Tony held out a small, flat, rounded stone that had the appearance of being held and rubbed often. He took my hand and put the little stone in it.

"Steve, this is a magic stone, I got it the last time I had an operation. If you hold the stone and close your eyes, you can travel to any place you want! It really works! And you can have it."

Tears leaked from the corners of my eyes, and my breath came in torn gasps. After a while, when I could contain myself, I thanked this incredible young man from the very bottom of my heart. I then looked over at Danny, and nothing needed to be spoken.

These two human titans took their good-byes and left.

I lay there thinking about life, how weird it is, and how lucky I was to have a friend like Danny Drazen.

New Growth

In the beginning a couple of my close friends would call daily, and at first I was so sick I really didn't want to talk much, just the call demonstrating their concern was comforting. Time passed slowly, and the longer I was in the hospital the fewer visitors came. That is just way things are, you have a catastrophe that feels like the end of the world, but the old world keeps on spinning outside the room. It was getting to be the middle of December, and I was worried about several things outside of my own strife.

My incredible wife was handling my sickness and still running the household. What choice did she really have when there is an eight year old and a fifteen year old to consider. I'm sure many people would have caved under such pressure. I knew her well enough to know how she internalized everything and wanted to please everyone, including me. So my concern was her stability.

Add to this smorgasbord of stress the Christmas crush. Presents for my family and hers, the kids, friends etc.

In the interest of trying to keep things normal as possible for the kids, these things had to go on un-interrupted. But I know the stress this caused Laura, and I was concerned.

The other huge item on my mind was my Mom. I had not seen her for a month. She was frail and sickly and I was really worried that I might never see her again. How long did I think even a failing elderly person was going to believe I had pneumonia?

One afternoon, as I lie in bed contemplating these things, a new doctor entered the room. I had heard he would be coming to see me.

"Hi, I'm Doctor Brown, and I'm a plastic surgeon. How are feeling?" he began.

"I thought I was just sick, not ugly!" I shot back, hoping to demonstrate the return of my good humor and get a chuckle. He seemed perplexed by that. I studied his face for a moment and realized it was not one that smiles sprouted from with any frequency. I was still too worn out to try and explain. A laugh wasn't that important to me.

"Your nurse reported that she observed some fresh new growth in your wound. I think we may be ready to close you up," was his good news for me. After he stated this I started to panic. Was he going to tear open the bandage from hell and pull the hated cotton out to look? I instinctively put my hand up to my chest as if to protect it from a sneak attack by this man.

"Does that mean that the infection is gone?" I inquired.

"It means that it is under control enough so that we can close the wound and treat it with antibiotics," the surgeon replied.

Encouraged, I gathered up the nerve to ask another question.

"Does that mean I can go home soon?" I ventured.

"It certainly moves you closer to that point, but you still have a ways to go," he answered, dousing my optimism with hard reality.

"In order to close you up," he pattered on as if discussing a recipe for spaghetti sauce, "we have to perform what is called a muscle flap. We need to get vasculated tissue into the wound, so you will heal properly."

I had no idea what he was talking about specifically, but the phrase 'muscle flap' had an ugly connotation.

"So Doc, what exactly does that mean?" I asked.

"As you know, the debreeding left you with a rather large crevice in your chest. All the wire and stitches, and a good amount of flesh and even some bone, had to be removed because of the infection. If I close you up like that, there won't be any tissue with veins in it to carry the antibiotic, which is distributed through the blood stream, to the infected area. A muscle flap is a procedure that replaces the debreeded area with muscle, which is vasculated tissue and so will carry the antibiotics where they are needed."

"Doc, I really hope to continue my life when this is all over, and lifting weights is a big part of that life. What does this mean, where are you going to get this vasculated tissue from?" I had visions of grafts and cuts and blood and I could feel my heart rate rising. You get focused on your heart rate in these circumstances.

"I plan to go up under your right arm."

He lifted up his own arm to demonstrate.

"I will detach your pectoral muscle right here and then turn the muscle, flipping it over, and lay it down in the crevice you have in your chest," he finished, seemingly pleased at his explanation of the procedure.

"So, let me get this straight," I countered, starting to get defensive and alarmed at the same time. "You want to cut my pectoral muscle from under my arm and replace my chest flesh with it?"

"Yes," was his hideous reply.

"What are my other options?" I asked, as if it was certain there were other options. I am always looking to make a counter offer or even suggest the obvious alternative that no one else but me can see.

"There aren't any," he stated, now sounding absolutely heinous to me.

"So, when does this next event take place?" I ventured.

"We have a room booked for tomorrow morning," he answered directly as he left. "Get some rest, you will feel better after we close that wound."

After lying there quietly absorbing the latest news, I started to actually get excited about the prospects of going home. I was looking forward to returning to normal. And I was looking forward to being able to see my mom.

Feeling well enough to care about returning to life, I called Laura to give her the good news. She was also excited; I could hear it in her voice.

Later that day, the nurses changed my dressing for the last time and I was whacked out on Morphine and Atavan. But through the fog I had the presence of mind to ask the nurse if I could see the anesthesiologist again. He was really busy and could not see me. However, I was able to communicate my wish to him to please remove the urinary catheter before I awoke from surgery.

CHAPTER EIGHT

My Chest Like A Roller Coaster

It never feels right or natural, awakening from surgery. This time awareness returned like ice out on one of the big lakes - all at once and you don't quite believe it. You can resist it, try to stay where it is warm and comfortable, but once you are awake you must finally surface. Even though waking up after surgery should have felt like old hat to me, the surprise was there.

After a quick check period in recovery, I was brought to my room.

A short while later, Laura arrived and I was so appreciative of her support. My wound was closed and my attention was focused on going home.

Later that same day Dr. Brown came in to see me. Several of the nurses and Physician Assistants had spoken highly of Dr. Brown. One nurse said she hoped that he would be my surgeon. Another let me know that he was hands down the best. Because of this, I had great confidence in him and therefore was not expecting what I was.

Knowing that I was somehow disfigured, but not sure to what extent, I was unprepared for his quick question, "Have you seen your wound yet?"

"Here we go again," I thought to myself as the nurse and Dr. Brown carefully undid the dressing on my newest wound.

When my chest had been revealed completely, all I could do was look and stare in disbelief.

I knew that my pectoral muscle was to be used, but what I saw was a series of hills like a roller-coaster ride starting from the top of my chest and, in a series of several mogul like bumps, ending just above my naval.

Cautiously, I looked at my right nipple. Dr. Brown had gone under my skin, under my nipple, and up to my right armpit to detach my main pectoral muscle. All my exterior skin was intact and normal looking. But down the middle were several mounds of flesh; all held together with staples that looked like something an industrial machine would use to close huge cartons. The mounds were my pectoral muscle, flipped over and laid down the middle of my chest where the crevice had been. The whole area was numb.

As I lay there looking at my new chest, Dr. Brown, who had been intently inspecting his work as though he had not seen it for weeks, asked, "How do you feel, I think this looks great!"

I honestly could not speak. I was conflicted between relief at being closed up and horror at my disfigured chest. I looked at him wanting to say something, but all I could do was look at him as tears ran down my face.

He seemed embarrassed by my tears.

"I can see you are upset, but all in all this looks very good and will heal well. A lot of this swelling will go down," he said as if apologizing.

I wanted to say, "It's OK doc, I know you did your best and that's just the way it has to be." But I honestly couldn't speak.

Continuing the visual journey of my redesigned chest, I noticed three tubes protruding from me. At the base of my incision, just above my naval, was one tube. It was connected at the end to a device that resembled a hand grenade, squished and sealed to create a vacuum. Visible inside the container was a collection of fluid, pinkish in color. Two other tubes extended from both my left and right sides, also ending in grenade type containers, squeezed and sealed to create the necessary vacuum. Pinkish fluid was being collected in these containers too.

Still somewhat numbed from all this new data, I looked in amazement at myself. Dr. Brown, seeing the attention I was giving to these tubes, explained their purpose.

"These tubes are creating a vacuum, holding everything in place while you heal. Since the wires have been removed from your chest, there is nothing to hold everything together. It is very important that you heal correctly. They will help you to drain better, which will speed up your recovery time."

I was trying not to think of the nightmare that pulling those tubes out would be. I was hoping they didn't go in that far, but of course I was fooling myself.

Exhausted by the whole ordeal, Laura left, once again solo, to see to the kids and house. She and the children were under huge stress. Now, at least, there was good news to tell Julie and Stevie at the dinner table. Daddy made it through his operation today!

The doctors and nurses went on about their busy schedules, and I fell back to sleep.

More Healing, One Step Closer To Home

The next day dawned bright and sunny and cold looking. I felt better just knowing I would not be facing the excruciating experience of having my chest ripped open twice that day.

I really was not in much pain. I had some discomfort (even I was using this metaphor for pain!) under my arm where the muscle was detached. The majority of my chest was just numb. I had no feeling at all in my right nipple. It was not the feeling you get when your foot falls asleep, it was just plain numb like a Novocaine shot.

About a week passed while my arm and chest healed. The nurses changed my grenades daily, carefully measuring the fluids, and squeezing the grenade tight every time. It was a cakewalk compared to the cotton baton form of torture!

I looked at my morphine pump.

"Time to get that thing out of here," I thought to myself. The last thing I wanted was to get addicted to that stuff. I had seen what that drug had done to some of my friends. When the nurse came in to bring the dreaded breakfast and inquire of my state, I asked that the pump be removed.

"Oh, you are going to want that for a while," was her prompt reply.

"But I don't think I need it," I stated. She looked at me like my Mother did when as a child I would say something foolish.

"You will be glad to have it for a while yet," was her admonishing prediction.

I proved her wrong. Over the next three or four days, several untouched, full cartridges of morphine were removed and new ones installed in my pump. I never used the device again.

Finally, as if it were the doctor's idea, the nurse announced the removal of my morphine pump. Its' departure was a small victory for me; "Just one step closer to home," was my thought.

Getting Closer

One morning Dr. Brown came in and broached the subject of tube removal. I was elated. The tubes were a big obstacle to getting out and going home.

"We will have to take these out one at a time," the good doc said. He meant one a day for three days. At least it was a time frame.

He grasped the tube and container from my left side gently and said "Here we go!" and it was out, painlessly. I was grateful and relieved.

The following day, Dr. Brown again visited me to remove the second tube. He decided to remove the center one, positioned right above my naval.

Once again, he gently took the tube in his hand and, with a "Here we go!" removed it. This time I could feel the depth the tube had penetrated. It felt like it was coming out from the center of my chest. In fact, it was. This is what he meant by "hold everything together." These tubes, by being connected to a vacuum, had kept my newly installed vasculated tissue, otherwise known as my pectoral muscle, firmly in place while healing occurred. To be effective they had to be quite a way in. It was not very painful, but very strange feeling. My optimism was returning, I could see light at the end of the tunnel.

Dr. Brown came in the next morning with his typical neutral expression. Soon, he was holding the last remaining tube in his hands. One more time, "Here we go!" and out came this last one. I could feel this one come out from under my arm! It was way in. The incision had been parallel to my naval. I had no knowledge of how invaded I had been! When the tube was out, he got right up and took everything into the bathroom, just as he had done previously. When he returned, I was still lying on my side, just trying to recover from the shock of having such a long tube removed from me.

"Are you all right?" he asked, somewhat concerned, I had not had a bad reaction from the previous two removals.

"Yeah, I'm fine," I lied. I was freaked out! I recovered quickly, thinking about going home. The good doctor checked a few more things and excused himself, he was satisfied with his work.

What's A Pick Line?

Several days later, as the calendar approached Christmas, a nurse I had not yet met came to see me. She explained that before I could go home she had been instructed to install a pick line in my arm for administering antibiotics. This all sounded swell.

"What exactly does that mean?" I inquired.

The nurse was examining my right arm, looking at veins and arteries, the expression on her face like a chess player choosing which piece to move.

"I am going to feed a small catheter into one of your veins that will go up your arm and almost to your heart. It will be parked in front of one of the major arteries feeding your heart. I will install an IV on this exposed end and you will be able to go home and administer antibiotics to yourself this way."

The going home part sounded like heaven, but the rest was just scary. After all the stuff that had already been done, I just accepted that this was the way it would have to be.

So, as I watched, she found a vein, and started the procedure. I had to look away as she threaded a small diameter catheter into my body.

When she was satisfied that all was in place, she left and an x-ray machine was wheeled into my room. The technician took a quick picture and left.

A short time later, my pick line nurse came back with the results of the x-ray.

"I thought you might like to see this," she stated.

The x-ray showed the line going into my chest and stopping just before my heart. The medicines would be released into my heart and distributed all throughout my blood system. This would hunt down any remaining infection and end it once and for all. And I could do this myself from the comfort of home sweet home!

The next day was December twenty second, and I was going home! I thanked my new found higher power; I would be home for Christmas.

Recovery would start again, and this time nothing could go wrong. My spirits soared and a feeling of hope that I had feared I would never sense again filled my heart.

CHAPTER NINE

Living With A Pick Line

This time I agreed willingly to a wheelchair ride to the front door. I was still a pretty sick guy, and needed help getting in and out of the chair.

Until everything healed, there really wasn't anything holding my chest together. I needed help getting in and out of the car, up from any chair, and in and out of bed. I learned to sort of tuck and roll to my side to get ready to be helped up, holding my arms to my chest to hold it all together.

At fifteen, my son Steve was as big as many men. His help was crucial. He could lift me as if I were a ninety-pound weakling! He never balked at putting his big arms around his once proud dad and helping me get up out of bed or of a chair. Still emotional from the surgery and drugs, I would try to hide my tears of pride and thanks for this young man who had grown so much while I was in the hospital.

Déjà vu. That was my thought as I attempted my first shower, with all the staples and hills and valleys that made up my chest.

My right arm, while not painful, wasn't much good yet. Before I could count on it for any help, the area under my arm where my pectoral muscle had been removed still had a good amount of healing to do.

As the warm water ran over my new/old wound, I was grateful again for being home. Everything in my house looked new to me. I was beginning to have this sense of a second chance, even though it really was my third!

In the hospital I had had plenty of time to reflect on life, and what I wanted from it. The 'every day is a bonus day' mentality that I now live with started to form concretely in my awareness those first few days home.

With help from Laura or Steve, I finished my shower and lay back down. After a brief rest, it was time for my first home injection. The only reason I was not apprehensive was because I had an IV line already installed, there would be no new punctures!

Sitting at the dinner table, Laura took out one of the syringes we had been given when we left the hospital. Unwrapping the IV, she stuck the end of the plastic syringe into the IV receiver. The directions instructed that it was necessary to take ten minutes to inject the entire syringe of antibiotic; it had to be absorbed over that time period. Every day, three times a day. But it was painless.

Soon it was time for Laura and Steve to get back to their daily schedules, Laura to teach school and Steve to attend his. So I was left to administer the antibiotics to myself, which I could do fine. But it was always nice when Laura got home and could help me.

The visiting nurses came several times a week. They dropped off supplies and generally checked me over. There were constant requests for my blood. I was convinced they were selling it!

Visiting Mom

On Christmas day I just had to see my Mom. She was doing all right in the nursing home, but was anxious to see me also. The last contact I had had with her was our wave on Thanksgiving Day!

After helping me perform all my morning activities, we packed up Laura's van and headed to the nursing home to see Mom. I was so excited and happy, it had been a month and a half since my heart attack, and I was thankful for this visit.

Laura's van died on the way to the nursing home! All I remember was how unreal it seemed. But we have a great neighbor, and Donny came to our rescue. He picked us up and drove us home to get my car.

We finally arrived at the nursing home and went directly to Mom's room. Both of us were so thrilled to see each other again!

I helped Mom into her wheelchair and wheeled her down to the lobby, as was our habit, to visit in a nice sunny spot.

All I could do was sob like a baby. My emotions just overran me. She looked at me, with a puzzled look on her face, and asked, "What are you crying about?"

I couldn't answer, but she knew it was because I loved her and had missed her. And as I sat there in the lobby of that nursing home, with the elderly and infirm all around, I looked at my Mother and my family and thanked my higher power for them, for my life and for a second chance. And I was determined to hold that focus for the rest of my life.

Return To Normal

For the next month and a half, I healed. During that time, I was allowed to call Jody in rehab at St. Joe's and get on a regular schedule. On my first day she greeted me like a long lost pal. She had heard all about my infection from Priscilla, my friend at the gym. While in the hospital I had stayed in touch with her by phone.

Feeling so much better, and being an impatient person, I was rearing to go. But the knowledgeable nurses in rehab slowed me down.

"You don't want to upset or tear your new grafts," they would admonish me when I would complain about not being allowed to run yet.

"You will get there, just work with us," Jody cajoled me.

The one factor that all the energy in the world can't control is time. And time is what it takes to heal. That point was made to me, and I had no desire to dispute their judgment.

Rehab was just exactly what I needed. It proved to me that I was getting better, and would get better.

Jody and her small circle of dedicated nurses were not used to having the patient push them. They were all great to me. There was Laurie, the pleasant brunette who seemed conservative in what she would let me do, but really knew how to help me not go over the limits. Kate was an Olympic Cyclist in training. Her workouts and races had taken her all over the world, and if medals were awarded on shear determination alone, she got the gold. Kate could relate to my need to regain the best part of myself, my health, my running.

But Jody was the center. She treated me like I was her personal friend. I guess I was. All her patients were.

Over time, my program of walking for ten minutes was increased to twenty. The nurses laughed at me. They were used to pushing their typically older patients do ten minutes! I was a square peg with a bunch of round holes all around me. At 47, I was by far the youngest patient.

One day, Jody came over to the treadmill I was walking on, a little faster than I thought she wanted me too, and said, "Go ahead and jog a little if you want."

With a grin you just couldn't wipe off my face, I moved the speed ahead and started jogging. Much sooner than I had anticipated, I was slowing the mill down and walking again.

Somewhat disappointed, I finished and as usual, went to cool down to have my blood pressure and heart rate checked.

"How did your jogging go?" Jody asked as another nurse took my reading.

"I guess I have a long way to go," was my negative reply. Jody could tell I was pretty disappointed.

"Steve, yes you do have a way to go, but that is what we are doing here. You should be encouraged!" Jody shot back.

Of course she was right! This made me smile, and after cooling down and getting ready to leave I told her, "I'll be back tomorrow and will run a little longer!"

"And a little longer every day after that!" She joined in.

And so it went, just as Jody had promised. I attended rehab four times a week and did some walking in between. I got stronger and stronger. My old self started to come back and I felt like the world was going to be OK.

I injected myself, or had help, three times a day and the visiting nurses gave me constant encouragement. The swelling did in fact go down on my chest, and the pectoral muscle that once graced my chest atrophied into the crevice that had been my sternum.

The staples came out and things started to get back to normal. Soon, my Infectious Disease Specialist, Dr. Stramphner, gave the OK for my pick line to come out. As a precaution, he put me on oral antibiotics. The line came out as painlessly as it went in, right in the convenience of my own home, at my own dinner table!

CHAPTER TEN

My Birthday Neck-ache

A bitter cold January passed and the cold month of February took its place. February is my birthday month, and I was thinking how lucky I would be to have another birthday!

On the fourteenth of February, Laura and I were attending a basketball game at one of the local elementary schools. My daughter Julie was playing, it was an Merrimack Youth Association game for the eight to ten year old girls.

She had improved greatly since I had last seen her play. What a terrific game! The only complaint I had was a pain in my neck. A pain that I just couldn't seem to shake. I asked Laura for some ibuprofen I knew she carried, and took three. They didn't touch the pain. I figured it must be a virus or something that had settled in my neck.

The next morning the pain seemed to be gone, but I noticed a reddening spot on my chest at the very top of my sternum; the top of my incision. It seemed slightly swollen, and my gut clenched like a fist. My old friend, denial, was right there for me. I knew I should call CMC and have the surgeons look at it, but I was desperately hoping it was something other than what I knew it to be.

Lurking on the outskirts of my mind, like an unwelcome quest at a picnic, was the truth. The infection was not dead. It was coming back with a vengeance!

Grasping at hope, I decided to call Jody at rehab. After describing the situation to her she asked me to come down to the hospital so that she could inspect my chest.

Jody took a brief look. Knowing full well what I had been through and how horrified I was at the prospect of the return of the infection, she looked at me with compassion and said, "Steve, I'm afraid you are having a relapse of the infection."

The Bring Your Own Dope Docs

She picked up the phone and called my primary doctor, sensing my reluctance to call the surgeons. Dr. Blackwood asked me to come right over. He wanted to look at the spot. He has been my doctor for many years and knew very well the emotional mess that I was becoming. He took one look and told his nurses to call CMC.

Earlier I mentioned that I had come to call my surgeons, the 'bring your own dope' docs. I was about to experience another episode!

The ride to CMC was a nightmare. Laura drove while I sat and moped. I was beside myself. I had accepted that my near death experience was over. There are three antibiotics that are effective against staff infection; three lines of defense. And if all three fail, you die.

I failed the first line when I had my initial surgery. It was standard operating procedure to administer antibiotics when you have open-heart surgery. But the antibiotics didn't prevent my first infection.

Since the infection had returned, I failed the second line of defense. That left one line of defense. I knew that much going into this visit. I had had many conversations during my visits with Dr. Stramphner, my Infectious Disease Specialist. He had very patiently explained these things to me.

My surgeon Dr. Brown met me in the emergency room. He explained that he would drain the walnut sized bump and install a wick. It sounded horrifying to me! He left to get prepped.

A wick, it turns out, is a piece of cloth left in a wound to keep it from healing over. In this case it was to let the pus drain.

Sitting on a bed in the emergency room was making me very upset, a bit edgy. The nurse on duty picked up on this and asked, "Would you be more comfortable in a private room?"

I jumped at her suggestion. The patients all around me were moaning and crying and starting to make me uncomfortable.

Still waiting for the doctor, the nurse had me follow her into an empty storage room! This was her idea of a private room. Laura and I could not believe our eyes, but it actually was better than listening to all the other patients in the main room. I was dealing with enough anxiety of my own!

Finally, Dr. Brown returned and inspected what was now a lump on my chest. He looked at it and explained that he was going to make a cut and expunge the puss and then install a wick. I asked about something for pain. He explained that pain pills were not that readily available. He had a new drug I could take orally that would be absorbed under my tongue and would dull the pain.

With a nurse assisting him, he made a cut in the swollen tissue forming the lump and together they squeezed the puss out. Then they installed a wick and covered the area up with a bandage. All of this was extremely uncomfortable, the under the tongue pill had done nothing.

"Where do we go from here, doc?" I asked, reluctant to hear the answer but knowing I must.

"You are going to have to be admitted and debreeded again" he replied. I knew that, but hearing it cut through me like a knife.

I Think I Know Her

They took me back to my old room. I was not nearly as sick as I had been during the previous stay in the "room reserved for the infected, the one in a hundred club," but there I was nonetheless.

The next morning, I went for my debreeding. Once again, there were discussions about urinary catheters, the ride to the OR, the waking up. Déjà vu!

Later that day I was lying in my room recovering. By now I knew lots of the faces and staff. Some I had become quite friendly with. I like to joke around and as I recovered during my earlier stays I had managed to have a few laughs with some of the staff.

Into my room came two nurses. One was a male nurse who had a similar sense of humor to me.

"Have you seen your wound?" was the familiar refrain. I was freaked out, but not as much as before. It actually seemed funny, in an ironic kind of way, to hear this being repeated to me.

Without waiting for an answer, the nurse started undoing my bandages. It seemed important to them to show me my new wound immediately after surgery.

When the bandages were removed, I looked down at my new wound. I had been reopened all the way down to my naval, and new industrial sized staples held the bottom two thirds of my wound together. The very top of my wound, where the red lump had been, was a debreeded hole in the top of my chest. It was red and shaped like a vagina. The RN and my friendly male nurse were watching me intently, serious expressions on their faces. It was an opportunity I couldn't resist.

"My God, I think I know her!" I spurted out.

The RN looked perplexed for a split moment, then briefly smiled before an admonishing, "Oh, stop!"

My friendly male nurse laughed out loud, heartily and without holding back. This earned him a dirty look from his female counterpart. Soon enough we were discussing the serious aspects of the wound and my comedic routine was forgotten.

A Short Stay

The next day I was already up and about, this surgery was much less debilitating than the previous two. I had recovered pretty well in rehab, jogging had definitely improved my stamina. So, even though I had been completely reopened, I was not ready to lie in bed.

Two days after my surgery, the pick-line nurse came to see me. I knew this meant I was going home again soon.

My new wound would require daily changing. The doctors explained how the nature of this wound was such that it would tunnel as it healed. The top part of the wound had suffered quite a bit of new bone and flesh loss. The nasty bugs had gotten into my bones! And they had gone quite deep. If this part closed up by healing over on the outside, it could cause a new infection, since it would leave a new breeding ground for the staff bugs in the warm, dark inside.

As the wound tried to close over on the outside, the way to keep it open and allow it to heal from the inside out, was to wick it. That meant that a piece of cotton strip would be inserted into the wound and changed daily. The visiting nurses would perform this rather unpleasant duty.

All of this was explained to me, the new pick line successfully installed, and I was rather unceremoniously discharged once again from CMC. I was now a senior member of the 'one in a hundred club'!

Back To Work

After a few days recuperating at home, I was ready to get back to my job of selling shipping supplies to manufacturers.

The July before my 'event' had occurred, I had joined a company and taken on a small local territory calling on manufacturers and other businesses that use boxes, tapes to close containers, strapping, stretch wrap for palletizing and other items that are regularly re-ordered. I had ventured out of the automotive industry for the first time in over twenty years.

"That business will give me a heart attack if I don't get out," I had told Laura.

My new boss, a great woman named Pat, had inspired me and I really gave the job all my attention and effort. I was landing new accounts at a pace of sometimes one or two a day! That I was headed for success was a sure bet.

When my heart attack hit, I was forced to stop all activities for Atlantic Shippers Supply. The business that I had generated continued to come in. Much to the credit of Atlantic Shippers, and something for which I will be eternally grateful to them, my commissions continued to be sent to the house. This was a real lifesaver!

Now I was intent on regaining my momentum. I started by working half days, the IV end of my pick line covered with a bandage. The nurse would come in the early morning and again in the late after noon. This allowed me to go out during the middle of the day.

Since the 'three times a day' self-injected antibiotic pick line system that I had used first failed, we were using an automatic pump that worked off and on all day. Every other day I needed to change the cartridges, which were supplied by the visiting nurses.

And so I sort of got back into the swing of things, but I never seemed to regain the drive I had naturally enjoyed. This seemed to perplex Pat and I know I caused her quite a bit of frustration. But she really believed in me, and kept encouraging me to try harder.

March, April and May came and went, and my wound got continually smaller. Soon it became necessary to use an ear swab to stuff the cotton strip into the small diameter hole that was still pretty deep. Keeping it open was a pain, but the risk of more infection was not something I was willing to consider.

Finally, one day the hole was too shallow to stuff anything into, and it healed over. All the doctors involved, including the one whose opinion I valued above all others, Dr. Stramphner, said it was time and I should be OK.

The pick line was out, and I was once again on oral antibiotics.

EPILOG

Out Of The Woods - Like It Never Happened

The rest of the story of my recovery seems a little anticlimactic after some of the trauma I experienced.

Laura and I met with an internationally acclaimed Cardio-thorathic surgeon who also is the leading professor of the same for Harvard University. My local doctor, a man of rare concern and interest in his clients, arranged an audience.

The surgeon/professor had reviewed all my records, which had been sent ahead, and highly praised the work the doctors at CMC had done on me. He further explained that the countrywide average for infections from open-heart surgery was three percent. That CMC had theirs down to one percent spoke extremely well of their staff (no pun intended!)

Laura and I left that interview convinced that the best that could have been done for me, was. I'll never know why the staff germs decided to go inward and try to eat me for dinner. All I can do is thank my higher power that I was able to get treatment, and be cured.

My life today, and how I live it, is like nothing ever happened. This is true to the extant that I do what I want, when I want, and in fact shovel snow just to prove that I can! I don't consider that I am a heart attack victim. I am a "still alive" winner. Talk about winning the lottery!

Anyone who is going through a similar ordeal is facing the reality of anticipating recovery with trepidation. But anything can be achieved with time and determination. The light at the end of the tunnel may seem faint and far away, but you will get there.

Fighting Denial

A recovering heart attack victim still has the same enemy to fight, denial! I try to remember, that each and every day is a bonus day for me. There is every reason to believe that I could have died that day. I knew something needing medical attention was occurring. After I had been able to accept the truth, I realized that a similar situation had presented itself a week or two earlier. I missed the warning because of denial.

The same feeling of having no energy, just flat spent, had come over me at the gym, even at the same time, right after a great workout. I took a sauna and a shower. I still felt poorly, but got dressed and headed up the highway to work. Even as it was happening, I knew I should have headed for the hospital. But, denial is a strong emotion. When, after a short distance to work, I felt better, like my old self, I just shook it all off and happily went on my way. Denial was better than facing reality. Heart problems don't happen to me!

What actually had occurred was a heart attack. I instinctively knew it, even though I had none of the regular symptoms. When the attack ended, and I felt like normal, I choose to ignore the event. What was I afraid of? Having my chest sliced open and my heart reworked? I was lucky. I had been experiencing cardiac arrest. Rather than deal with it, as I should have, I just ignored my problem.

In the emergency room Dr. Liebling told me that I might die, that there was a good chance I wouldn't survive the attack. Would he have said the same thing a week earlier? I'll never know, but the fact that I got a second chance, and lived to take advantage of it, had to be related to my exercise program.

I live life like every day is one I might not have had if I lived twenty years earlier. We have medical and social perks that our ancestors could not have dreamt of. And still, people like me would rather go into denial than make use of our benefits.

Collateral Damage

It is important to understand the affect of a heart attack victims' illness on others. Those others will almost definitely include family members, and can extend to friends, neighbors and certainly people with whom you work.

So, how does your illness affect these relationships? I can tell you how my situation affected my family.

Steve Jr., my first born, was fifteen when disaster struck. Fifteen is such a dynamic age for a young man. Many impressionable ideas are taking form during those years and Dad and Mom are so important.

When the first part of my episode hit, I said to Steve, "Honey, I'm not trying to put extra stress on you, but right now, you are going to have to be the man of the family and help your Mom and sister out as best you can. The best way for you to do that is to do the things you need to do for yourself, and be there for the girls. I'll be getting better and will be home, but I am thankful to know I can rely on you."

Steve responded with the bravado and strength that I had expected. He had always been a loving and responsive child, now he was showing his maturity. He was strong and supportive from start to the finish when I was finally out of the hospital.

During my whole illness, I had been on an emotional roller coaster. Imagine what it must have been like for a fifteen-year-old boy. Not knowing from one day to the next whether or not your father was going to live. On the days that seemed bad, I'm sure thoughts such as, "Who will take care of us?" and "Will my Dad die?" went through his head.

When things seemed to be OK after my first surgery, I'm sure he was relieved, only to be blasted again by my first infection and return to the hospital. Then after several months of recuperation, another plunge down when my second infection returned and I was on my last line of defense.

He was forced to deal with not one catastrophe but several successive ones. He pulled his weight and everything seemed OK.

A month or two after my last episode, the four of us were having dinner one night as usual. Laura noticed a few odd looking scratches on Steve's arm.

"What are those marks?" Laura, ever the alert teacher asked.

"Oh, nothing," came the typical fifteen year old answer.

But "oh nothing" does not fly with Laura. She continued to press, insisting he pull his sleeve up further. When he did, it revealed several more small marks, cuts, actually, as it turned out. Perceptive and now alarmed, Laura dug some more and discovered that Steve had been making small cuts on his arm. She correctly identified this as a sign of disturbance, and quickly made arrangements for professional help.

For the next six months or so Steve received counseling and responded to it very well, eventually dealing with his feelings and moving forward with his life. Thanks to Laura, Steve has been back to his old self for four years. Fortunately she knew how to address the situation and we found a professional who could help.

Julie, a third grade student at the time, was told, "Dad will be all right" and was young enough to just accept that. She never really demonstrated any type of disturbance from the experience. With the writing of this book, Julie is finally coming to understand the severity of the illness I experienced.

Laura was the rock of Gibraltar during the entire experience. I have written of my concern for her, how the stress of a seriously ill spouse coupled with the huge responsibility of being a working mom would take its toll. But she seemed to get through it all, holding up like an oak.

About a month or so after all was declared well, one evening in the middle of the night I awoke to find her out in the living room walking around, wide eyed and looking really wired. A quick check of her heart rate was 120, well over the safe zone!

The next morning I called in sick and we headed for the local emergency room. Once there, she was diagnosed as having panic attacks and was medicated accordingly. The effects of all the stress and responsibility of keeping things as calm and normal for the sake of the kids had finally come home to roost. It is an amazing phenomenon, the way she was able to hold her feelings in. Once I was out of the water, her psyche finally allowed her to release her fears and worries. These were manifest in this physical condition typical of too much stress and anxiety.

As time went on and our lives got back to normal, Laura got back to her old self and she too has been fine.

Thanks For Listening!

Try to live in the moment. Stay in the moment. I need to remember every day, in the style of Buddhist teachings, that if we are worried about tomorrow, we are not living in the right now. If we are thinking about a lost opportunity from yesterday, today is slipping by un-lived! When I am able to focus on living in the moment, problems and chores become smaller, they start to fit in with the right now I am focused on! My stress level is lessened.

It is not easy to focus on right now. We have a natural tendency to worry about tomorrow or yesterday. But we are wasting our lives doing so.

As of this writing, I have been infection free for almost five years. I don't expect the infection to ever return, but I also know that medical professionals don't know everything.

And my life style is not always perfect, either. There are periods when I forget that I have heart disease, and I eat poorly.

I am fortunate that I am able to stay focused on my exercise program, but even that goes up and down. I recently had to loose about twenty pounds. I had let my running go a little over the winter, and had not watched my weight.

But, I am fighting my continuing denial! I'm back on track, paying the price with sore legs and shorter runs than I would like to do. But I'll get back to where I can run a few miles. I lift five days a week, and really enjoy that more. It is more social, and I enjoy my friends at the gym.

I hope to see you there!

www.ingramcontent.com/pod-product-compliance
Lightning Source LLC
Chambersburg PA
CBHW080435290526
45791CB00008BA/2506